THE FIRST YEAR™

Lupus

An Essential Guide for the Newly Diagnosed

NANCY C. HANGER is a freelance writer and editor living in New Hampshire, with a husband, three cats, and over 10,000 books in a renovated farmhouse and barn named Windhaven. She coauthored *Essential Business Tactics for the Net* (Wiley, 1998), and is a columnist for BYTE.com and WIRED News, but has always fallen back on her first love: editing and developing books. She has been editing primarily in the science fiction and genre fiction fields since the 1980s. After being diagnosed with lupus-related conditions in the early 1990s, she tried cutting back on her fulltime work, but found she only filled in with more hobbies, including knitting, weaving, and spinning. Her freelance business, Windhaven Press, handles book editing and production for most of the major publishing houses in New York.

THE COMPLETE FIRST YEAR™ SERIES

THE FIRST YEAR™

Lupus

An Essential Guide for the Newly Diagnosed

Nancy C. Hanger

Foreword by Andrea B. Schneebaum, M.D.

IPANY ■ NEW YORK

Published by
Marlowe & Company
An Imprint of Avalon Publishing Group Incorporated
161 William Street, 16th Floor
New York, NY 10038

Library of Congress Cataloging-in-Publication Data
is available.

ISBN 1-56924-509-6

9   8   7   6   5   4   3   2   1

Designed by Pauline Neuwirth,
  Neuwirth and Associates, Inc.

Printed in the United States of America

Distributed by Publishers Group West

To my husband, Andrew, who puts up with me daily,
and to my parents, who taught me to be the strongest woman
I could be.

Thanks, all of you, for letting me know that it's okay to be a "sick
broad."

Pain is real when you get other people to believe in it. If no one believes in it but you, your pain is [presumed to be] madness or hysteria.

—Naomi Wolf, *The Beauty Myth*

Contents

Contents

Foreword

by Andrea B. Schneebaum, M.D.

SYSTEMIC LUPUS ERYTHEMATOSUS (SLE) is considered the hallmark of systemic autoimmunity and challenges the clinician with its diversity. Research has progressed enormously in the last decade. Serologic markers have been identified to help in diagnosis, as predictors of specific organ/system involvement and as indicators of disease activity. Newer, more specialized drugs that can target cell messages or specific antibody production are being tested and used to treat various aspects of SLE. It is an exciting time to be a rheumatologist.

Yet, as a clinician, I am often humbled by the strength of will that my patients exhibit to just get through their days. While many do not suffer from the medically severe aspects of SLE—recurrent strokes, severe heart or lung disease, or kidney failure—they deal with chronic fatigue, vague yet intense pain, and loss of mental concentration and acuity.

The hardest aspects of SLE and many chronic illnesses are addressed in this book. I agree that being able to differentiate the cause of a particular symptom is critical, but as a physician I am frustrated by the paucity of tools I have to solve some of these problems.

Nancy Hanger presents a mind-set that is practical and encouraging. She offers personal accounts that add reality to her words. She hits upon the key ingredient for success—education—and helps her readers to find for themselves the appropriate support groups—medical specialists, family, and friends—and directs readers to appropriate on-line resources. She helps her readers define for themselves their own parameters of stress and fatigue. She then helps them catalogue this information so that they can make useful and practical decisions that can empower them to accomplish their own goals. She sets an example through her own work of how we can all be successful.

This book is a first step in learning about SLE as a chronic illness. I cannot emphasize enough how much more we all need to learn.

ANDREA B. SCHNEEBAUM, M.D., completed her specialty training in rheumatology at the University of Colorado Health Sciences Center in Denver, with both research and clinical training in autoantibody production and SLE. After practicing at the Lahey Clinic in Burlington, Massachusetts, and participating on the board of the Massachusetts chapter of the Lupus Foundation for over ten years, she and her family moved to southern New Hampshire, where she works as a clinical rheumatologist.

Introduction

IF YOU'RE reading this book, chances are you or someone you know has been diagnosed with lupus. This book is designed to bring you information to help alleviate some of the fears you may have about lupus, answer some of the questions that are probably topmost in your mind, and help you approach it as a disease that can be handled daily and lived with for many years to come.

Receiving a diagnosis of lupus is scary—there's no question that it can be an overwhelming pronouncement. Take a deep breath and step back. This book is here to aid you in your journey through the first year of having lupus: you have a companion in your travels, now.

No one knows what causes lupus, though it is suspected that there is a genetic link of predisposition to getting the disease. *Lupus* is a rheumatological, autoimmune disease affecting the entire body's connective tissues: muscles, tendons, skin, blood, organs, and connective linings. It is related to rheumatoid arthritis, but unlike arthritis, it can endanger the patient because of the way it attacks the body's systems. Lupus is not a disease that can be cured at this time.

Lupus is, in a nutshell, a disease that attacks your own body out of confusion. Lupus makes your body think that perfectly good parts of it are "wrong," then attacks them as if they need to be fixed, which means you end up with inflammation in places that would otherwise be left alone. You can end up with anything from tendonitis to pericarditis (inflammation of the sac surrounding the heart) to pneumonia to blood clots.

Lupus comes and goes. It is a disease that goes into remission, sometimes for many years, only to reappear out of the blue. No one knows what makes it do this, but it does seem to be mostly related to stress. Because of that, this book will also talk about handling your stress levels and how you can lower your stress in order to make the lupus go into remission more readily.

How this book is organized

I have written this book as if you have just been diagnosed with lupus and are about to embark on your first full year post-diagnosis with the disease. Each section is divided into days, weeks, and months, taking you through the first week, day by day; the first month, week by week; and the rest of the first year, month by month. At each section break we will look back at what you've learned, lived through, and look forward to in your journey.

The chapters of this book are divided into two sections: Living and Learning. In the Living sections, you will discover ways in which lupus is handled on a daily basis, how you can live with various syndromes associated with lupus, overlapping conditions, medications that may be prescribed for you during the course of the disease, and other aspects of your life that will most likely be affected by lupus over the course of a year. The Learning sections go into more depth concerning information about lupus conditions, medications, prognosis, therapies, research into the disease, and medical details about lupus and associated overlapping syndromes.

Some terms in this book will show up in **boldface**. This means these words are defined in more detail within the glossary located on page 229.

By the end of this book, you will have lived a full year with lupus, experiencing and learning about many of its aspects, conditions, and treatments. You will be armed with the knowledge and assurance that *living* with lupus is not only possible but something that *you* can do every day, throughout your life.

Finally, this book is interactive. I have included some worksheets and exercises to help you address some of the issues that appear to cause lupus "flares" (when lupus becomes more active), so you can reduce the times that lupus can interfere in your life.

Why I wrote this book

About nine or ten years ago, I started to become quite ill. I had rotating bouts of tendonitis that were incapacitating for me—tendons in my arms, my legs, my back, all over, would suddenly become inflamed, hurt like the devil for weeks at a time, then subside again as mysteriously. It would move around, almost as if it were alive: first my arms would have it, then it would suddenly move to my legs. It was a mystery to everyone, and frustrating to my doctors, who finally ended up trying to track it as if it were a histrionic (emotional) reaction I was causing myself. After all, my job in book editing and production can be a stressful one. I remained skeptical: I knew my body was up to something. But what?

I became exhausted, almost unable to work, which caused more stress in my life. I began to question whether the doctors were right, after all: Was this all in my mind?

After about a year of this, my general practitioner of the time (who was also, coincidentally, one of my karate instructors), started mentioning the word "lupus." Thus started my journey toward discovering what lupus was, what it could do to the human body, and how in the world people could live with such a disease.

Since then, I have been rediagnosed with lupus, undiagnosed by another doctor, rediagnosed by yet another doctor, and undiagnosed by a fourth. Lupus is like that: it can be a frustrating disease to live with—it's hard to pin down, sometimes. There are blood tests (such as the ANA, a rheumatoid factor) to define it, but some people fall outside the curve that the blood tests measure (non-ANA lupus comprises a distinct percentage of lupus patients worldwide, and the number continues to rise). Some doctors don't think that "non-ANA lupus" exists, so many patients continue to go undiagnosed, while others are treated *as if* they have lupus, but remain unlabelled in the medical system.

In the last several years, I have been diagnosed with two of the major overlapping syndromes associated with lupus: Sjögren's Syndrome and Raynaud's Syndrome, both of which cause inflammatory and auto-immune responses, just like lupus. Because of Sjögren's Syndrome, I have to carry a water bottle and eye drops with me at all times—my body is no longer capable of producing adequate saliva and tear film, and I can literally dry up to a painful and dangerous extent. Because of Raynaud's Syndrome, I have had one blood clot in my left leg, landing me in the hospital right in the middle of a book production deadline. The nurses at the hospital had to forcibly remove book page proofs from my hands to make me take a nap! Raynaud's also means I have to wear socks and gloves to bed; my hands and feet are so cold, I often can't fall asleep (not to mention the comments I get about my "popsicle toes" from my husband, Andrew!).

I'm not complaining about my life, though. It's livable, and enjoyable, in spite of all these syndromes. At times, my friends and family laugh about it. My friend Bruce makes fun of me—almost daily—about how clumsy I've become because of the peripheral neuropathy I have in my left foot. "But I used to be a ballet dancer!" I'll shoot back, after he rolls his eyes—yet again—when I stumble over my own feet on my driveway. We both laugh and make jokes about me needing kneepads just to walk around the house. If you don't laugh at yourself, who will? After all, you can laugh at yourself much better than anyone else can.

Lupus isn't the end of life. Living with it is your job now, and like any job, sometimes it can be an easy one and sometimes it can be more difficult. This book is designed to help you find some answers when living with lupus seems confusing and difficult. I hope I've succeeded in making your "job" a bit easier.

Twelve-step groups have coined the phrase "one day at a time." That's what living with lupus can often be like. But if you take the small, daily steps necessary, approaching lupus isn't quite as overwhelming as you may think.

This book will not prescribe

While I have chapters here that discuss some of the medications and therapies commonly prescribed for lupus patients, this book will not recommend medication nor will it prescribe medication for you.

Only you and your doctor can determine what medications are best for you at any given time. Lupus is a disease that has several base conditions, but it also has many overlapping conditions that can present themselves at any time—no one knows what conditions will show up for you, and no one can predict if any one condition will *ever* be present in your case. Your doctor will treat these conditions as they arise.

Never take any medication, herbal remedy, or therapy without consulting your rheumatologist or primary care physician first. This is very important. Medications all affect one another, and even a "simple herb" can be dangerous if taken in conjunction with another certain herb or medication. Only your doctor, who is professionally trained in prescribing medications, can tell you what you should take, with what, and when.

The same goes for therapies: do not start any kind of therapy, even a nontraditional one, without consulting with your physician first. If you feel uncomfortable talking to your doctor about nontraditional therapies and wish to "hide" that from him or her, it's time to either reconsider how you interact with your physician, or find a physician you feel more comfortable talking to about these things. *Never **not** talk* to your doctor about anything you want to do in the form of therapy or medication.

Because lupus is an autoimmune disease, your body is already confused enough, trying to sort out what to "attack" and what to leave alone. Taking medication without a proper prescription could lead to a fatal condition—give your body a break and always talk to your doctor.

Keep on learning about lupus

This book is only a jumping-off point for you. Your journey with lupus will continue for the rest of your life. Learn as much as you can about lupus from reputable sources—one of the chapters here talks about how to find such places. In the back of this book you will find resources to write to and Web pages to visit that can help you with your research in the future. Take advantage of the information from such places as the Lupus Foundation of America. Find support groups in your area—the information they will supply, and the support they can give during difficult times, could prove invaluable during your lifetime with lupus.

No one knows what causes lupus, to this day. Researchers have their suspicions, and research is being done in many fields, including genetics and recombinant DNA work. The fact remains, however, that much work is yet to be done before a "cure" for lupus can ever be found. First we need to know where it comes from and why. Future research will probably give us a reason why lupus arises, and perhaps eventually a cure can be found, but that's likely a long way off. Supporting such research is important: groups like the Lupus Foundation of America help fund research into lupus. Check out the LFA as well as other reputable lupus foundations to see how you, your friends, and your family can help.

In the meantime, learn as much as you can about your disease, because knowledge is indeed power. The more you know, the more you will be able to control the flare-ups of lupus, and the easier it will be for you to live an active lifestyle. *Living with* lupus is your goal: you can learn to control your disease to a degree, through stress reduction, learning your triggers (what causes lupus to flare up for you), and managing your medications and therapies with your doctor.

Don't be afraid to learn as much as possible about lupus. Armed with that knowledge, you can help others who have been newly diagnosed—let them know, as I will in this book, that they are not alone. Lupus may be a scary diagnosis, but we can live with it and laugh at the funny bits and help each other along the way.

Support is very important for lupus patients: I hope this book will be a support for you in the first year you have lupus. Let's take that journey together.

Nancy C. Hanger
Auburn, New Hampshire
July 2003

THE FIRST YEAR™

Lupus

An Essential Guide for the Newly Diagnosed

Diagnosis— At Last

YOU'VE JUST gotten a diagnosis from the doctor that you have Systemic Lupus Erythematosus (SLE). Most likely, you have been seeking a diagnosis of some sort for quite a while. It's not unusual for lupus patients to go undiagnosed for up to ten or fifteen years, while others are diagnosed right away. If you're in the group of those who have had to wait for a diagnosis, rest assured that you're not alone. Neither are you alone if you feel you have been undergoing a frustrating and overly long journey toward this diagnosis: lupus, as with many of the **autoimmune diseases,** is one of the "great imitators." Many other diseases look and act like lupus's symptoms; don't be angry if your doctor has misdiagnosed many other diseases on his way to diagnosing you with lupus—this is normal.

It's also normal to be frightened when hearing the diagnosis: after all, lupus has had a reputation for being a scary disease. Hang in there and read further. While lupus can be a serious disease, it's not necessarily fatal, nor is there anything to be scared of once you have educated yourself about this illness.

You feel relieved

It's been a long road getting a diagnosis of lupus. You've now made it through what may be the most difficult part of the process: getting a definitive diagnosis. Feeling relief isn't bad—it's normal. We are all conditioned to think that getting a diagnosis of a serious disease isn't something one should feel relief about; you're probably having conflicting thoughts on why you feel relief, and you possibly have some guilt associated with these feelings. This is also normal—just about all lupus patients go through this. If you are a woman, these feelings may be compounded. This is primarily a "**woman's disease**," and many conflicting emotions about why you have lupus, how you got it, and why it was so difficult to diagnose are going to surface from all concerned: from you, your doctor(s), your friends, and family.

You may want to talk to your doctor about these feelings, as well as your family and friends. You may want to explain to them that the long process of getting a diagnosis has been as difficult for you as it has for them, and that you feel relieved that a diagnosis has been made—not that you necessarily feel relief that you have the lupus itself. Open communication is very important with lupus; it will help you in the future as the disease develops and you go through various cycles of **flaring** and **remission**, as you seek support from your doctors and family/friends.

It's not all in your head

Your diagnosis assures you that what you've been experiencing as symptoms and illnesses is *not* "all in your head." It's likely that at one point someone told you that you have exaggerated or even made up your symptoms: this is very common with lupus. Everyone in my lupus support group, Wolfbytes, has had this said to them, often more than once. We compare stories each time one of us runs into yet another physician who utters the words, "It's all in your head" or "I know you *think* you're sick, *but* ..." or (our personal favorite) "Maybe you're just a little depressed." If you've heard these words, we sympathize with you: you're not alone.

It's a very difficult disease to diagnose at first, and because it affects primarily women, the symptoms are often dismissed as secondary to depression or even hypochondria. You now know that it's not your fault and it's not something you made up: you have a real disease that has a name, classified symptoms, bona fide support groups and national organizations.

Lupus is a more widespread disease than most people think. The National Lupus Foundation of America estimates that 16,000 Americans develop lupus every year and 500,000 to 1.5 million Americans have been diagnosed with the disease. Eight to ten times more women than men develop lupus, and women of non-Caucasian ethnicity are affected more highly (and develop it later in life and go undiagnosed longer). As yet, no one knows why this is so, but the National Institute of Arthritis and Musculoskeletal and Skin Diseases (NIAMS), as part of its strategic plan for reducing health disparities, is researching this area.

Lupus isn't always fatal

It's scary to receive a diagnosis of lupus: soap operas and other popular entertainments often portray people with lupus as having a "fatal disease," replete with dramatic deathbed scenes. While that may have had a grain of truth as little as twenty years ago, it simply isn't true anymore.

When it was first suggested to me by my then primary care physician that I had lupus, I told one of my good friends, Bruce, about the news. The first words out of his mouth, after he paused to think, were "So you're going to die." Another friend, Mark, said, "I don't know if I can handle that." To both of them, I had to explain that lupus wasn't necessarily fatal: that I had a greater chance of being hit by a truck (and I live on a rural, residential street). Both of their reactions are quite typical—the general public still views lupus as something (1) people get if they live in a soap opera on TV, and (2) something that kills you fast and nastily. Luckily, neither of those views are correct, and I was able to assure my good friends that I was probably going to get sick more often than normal, but I wasn't going to die.

While lupus is a serious disease, it is *not* necessarily fatal. Eighty to ninety percent of lupus patients survive their first ten years after diagnosis and go on to live full lives. Diagnosis of lupus has improved a hundredfold in the last twenty years, particularly with the advent of blood test diagnoses such as the rheumatoid factor (ANA) and others, leading to earlier diagnosis and therefore earlier treatment. Treatment has also improved, adding nonsteroidal anti-inflammatories (**NSAIDs**) and various sophisticated yet gentle chemotherapies to the arsenal in the last twenty years.

Having lupus means *living with lupus*. This is not the time to give up and decide that the diagnosis means you have something you can't live with and can't fight. That's nonsense: lupus is eminently treatable and thousands live with the disease until old age. This is the time for you to educate yourself as much as you can about your disease and decide that *living* with lupus is your positive answer to your diagnosis.

IN A SENTENCE:

> *Diagnosis of systemic lupus is scary, but living with it is possible and can be a positive experience.*

learning

What is Lupus?

LEARNING WHAT lupus is, and isn't, is key to learning to live with it. In this section we will learn what systemic lupus erythematosus is, what its causes may be, its symptoms, a checklist to diagnose lupus, what other forms of lupus there are, and why lupus is often called a "mimicking" disease.

What is SLE?

Systemic Lupus Erythematosus (SLE), which we will refer to simply as *lupus* in this book, is a **rheumatological** and autoimmune disease affecting the entire bodily system. It primarily affects the pulmonary system (lungs and blood circulation), heart, joints, kidneys, and skin. The immune system is what keeps us healthy—immune antibodies attack disease. In the case of lupus, the immune system becomes confused and the antibodies attack healthy tissue and organs, creating symptoms that range from skin rashes to inflammation in the heart or kidneys. Most often, lupus patients have joint problems, as lupus is a rheumatological disease affecting the connective tissues (joints, muscles, and organs), and can be treated along with rheumatoid arthritis.

Lupus is also often categorized as a diffuse **connective tissue** disease. A connective tissue disease is anything that affects the connective tissue in the body: muscles, tendons, organs, and other connecting tissues.

What causes lupus?

No one knows definitively what causes lupus. Many researchers today are working on finding a genetic cause of lupus, and in fact recently (1997, National Institute of Health News Release) researchers reported in the *Journal of Clinical Investigation* that they found a "lupus gene" on chromosome 1. What this means to lupus patients is unclear, however; it could be that lupus can be passed along genetically in family lines, but it also could mean that one of these genes on chromosome 1 can get *damaged,* causing lupus to develop in the patient. It is also unclear because lupus, like rheumatoid arthritis, is a *complex genetic* disease, meaning one gene may link to a predisposition to develop lupus, but other genes must interact with that gene plus an external factor (such as environmental exposure, like chemicals or sunlight) to trigger the lupus itself. Research on chromosome 6 was done in the past, also linking lupus to a genetic predisposition.

All this said, according to the Lupus Foundation of America, only ten percent of lupus patients will have a direct family member who also has lupus. This means much more research into the causes of lupus, and all rheumatological diseases, must continue.

As stated before, about ten times more women than men develop lupus, causing researchers to wonder if there is an estrogen (female hormone) component involved in lupus; many women develop lupus in their early twenties, after completing their full growth. Research into this area has much more work to go before anything definitive can be stated.

The same goes for ethnic selection: for reasons unknown, it appears from statistics that more African-American, American-Indian, Latino, and Asian women suffer from lupus than Caucasian. Research in this area continues, particularly along the lines of inequalities in health care, living conditions (with the possibilities of environmental contaminants as a factor in damaging these women's genetic structures), and overall availability of early diagnosis for these ethnic groups.

Lupus can also be caused by exposure to certain drugs (especially the sulfa and penicillin antibiotics) and hormones (in which case it is referred to as **drug-induced lupus**), and by stress and ultraviolet light. Some cases of lupus appear to be triggered by exposure to certain other diseases and infections.

What does this all mean? No one knows for sure exactly how any one case of lupus has been caused.

What are the symptoms of lupus?

Lupus has a large number of symptoms, but the most common, according to the Lupus Foundation of America and other lupus foundation sources are:

- ○ Achy or swollen joints
- ○ Frequent fevers (over 100 degrees F)
- ○ Arthritis
- ○ Muscle weakness and aches
- ○ Migraines (headaches)
- ○ Peripheral neuropathy (tingling feet and hands)
- ○ Fatigue (prolonged or excessive)
- ○ Skin rashes (usually caused by sunlight exposure)
- ○ Anemia
- ○ Kidney problems
- ○ **Pleurisy** (painful breathing)
- ○ **Malar rash** (the "butterfly" rash across the cheeks and nose)
- ○ Sun and ultraviolet light sensitivity

○ Hair loss
○ Blood clotting problems
○ Fingers turn blue or white from cold exposure (**Raynaud's Syndrome**)
○ Seizures
○ Mouth or nose ulcers

Some or all of these symptoms may occur while you have lupus. Not all people develop all symptoms, and some people develop symptoms and complementary diseases and syndromes on their own. When you have other syndromes and diseases along with lupus, it is referred to as **overlapping lupus**.

There is a standard checklist from the American College of Rheumatology (ACR), issued in 1982, of symptoms and tests to diagnose lupus: the sidebar on this page lists these for you. Note that this checklist is due for updating, and many other physicians, particularly in England, have been coming up with their own alternative checklists (see Suggested Reading in the appendices). From this ACR checklist, you must have four or more of these symptoms in order for a diagnosis of lupus to be positive. Be aware that this list is used primarily for statistical research purposes.

Other kinds of lupus

SLE is only one type of lupus, though it covers many of the other types within itself. There are four basic other types of lupus erythematosus: discoid, drug-induced, neonatal, and overlapping.

DISCOID LUPUS

Discoid or **cutaneous** lupus primarily affects the epidermis or skin. This is the most common type, second only to joint pain as a symptom in common LE. Discoid or chronic cutaneous LE, subcutaneous LE, and acute cutaneous LE are the three primary types of skin lupus. There are other types of skin lesions that affect people with lupus, but which also occur in other diseases, such as vasculitis (problems with blood flow), calcinosis (calcium deposits in the skin), hair loss, and

Symptom Checklist

Malar Rash	Rash over cheeks and nose, in a "butterfly" pattern
Discoid Rash	Raised red patches, often on the arms and upper arms
Photosensitivity	Reaction to sunlight or ultraviolet light, usually as a skin rash
Oral ulcers	Painless (usually) ulcers in mouth and/or nose
Arthritis	Nonerosive (joints do not deteriorate) arthritis in two or more peripheral joints
Serositis	Pleuritis (inflammation of the pleural lining around the lungs) or pericarditis (inflammation of the lining around the heart)
Renal disorder	Excessive protein in the urine and/or abnormal elements derived from red and/or white cells and/or kidney tubule cells
Neurologic disorder	Seizures and/or psychosis in the absence of drugs or metabolic disturbances
Hematologic disorder	Hemolytic anemia or leukopenia (low white blood count) or lymphopenia or thrombocytopenia (in the absence of drugs or other disturbances). The leukopenia and lymphopenia must be detected twice or more.
Antinuclear antibody	Positive test for antinuclear antibody (ANA) in the absence of drugs that can cause it
Immunologic disorder	Positive, anti-double stranded anti-DNA test, positive anti-Sm test, positive antiphospholipid antibody such as anticardiolipin, or false positive syphilis test (VDRL)

Note that the false positive syphilis test used to be one of the primary ways of testing for lupus twenty years ago.

(Adapted from Tan, E.M., et al., *The 1982 Revised Criteria for the Classification of SLE. Arth Rheum* 25:1271-1277, 1997 revision.)

Raynaud's Syndrome (fingers and toes turn blue or white in the cold). People who have discoid lupus often never develop systemic lupus, while others will go on to eventually develop it. While having discoid LE, it's common for patients to not test positive for ANA factors in the blood and other common SLE blood tests.

Drug-induced lupus

Drug-induced lupus is literally just that: a drug taken for another disease or illness causes lupus to develop. According to Robert L. Rubin, Ph.D., of the Scripps Research Institute, at least 38 different medicines can cause lupus after being taken for prolonged periods, including medicines for heart disease, thyroid disease, hypertension, neuropsychiatric disorders and some anti-inflammatory agents and antibiotics (particularly the sulfa derivatives and penicillin). The three most prevalent drugs related to drug-induced lupus are:

- procainamide (Pronestyl)
- hydralazine (Apresoline)
- quinidine (Quinaglute)

It takes at least several months of continual use for any drug-induced reaction to occur, and those who already have SLE do not show any proclivity to develop more symptoms of lupus from taking those drugs.

No one knows what causes drug-induced lupus or why some people get it and others don't while taking the same drugs. Some research focuses on how drugs metabolize in the body, others focus on multiple processes and how they interact with not only the drug itself but how the immune system interacts with it. Links between how "normal" SLE develops and how drug-induced lupus develops are being researched now.

Neonatal lupus

Neonatal lupus is the third type of lupus, and is a bit of a misnomer. Neonatal is a very rare condition and is not at all the same thing as SLE. It affects newborns who acquire maternal (from the mother) autoantibodies that affect the heart, skin, and blood. There is also a photo-sensitive rash that appears during the first few weeks of the newborn's life, which may persist for several months.

OVERLAPPING LUPUS

Lupus does not usually occur in a vacuum. Most people with SLE have overlapping diseases and syndromes, many of which we will discuss later in this book during Day Six and Months Three, Four, and Five. Because of all these overlapping syndromes, lupus is a complicated disease—another reason why it is so difficult to diagnose.

Why is lupus so hard to diagnose?

Lupus is one of the great mimicking diseases, akin to Multiple Sclerosis (MS) in that way (though they are very different diseases!). Lupus can, at times, appear to be anything from chronic migraines to simple gastrointestinal disorders (such as irritable bowel syndrome) to chronic fatigue syndrome to fibromyalgia to dermatitis—anything that can be a symptom or a distinct syndrome can be interpreted as its own disease, and often is. With lupus acting as an overlapping disease in anywhere from five to thirty percent of diagnosed patients, you can only imagine what a nightmare diagnosis can be for some doctors.

While I was waiting for my own diagnosis, I often got frustrated with all the difficulties inherent in the overlapping syndromes and symptoms. I know from correspondence with many other people with SLE that they have experienced just as much or even more frustration than I. I got to the point where I gave up wanting to know what the disease I had was called: I called it "Fred." What the heck, Fred was Fred and at some point he would have a formal name—for the time being, I was caught up in simply trying to *live* with all the symptoms and syndromes. And live I did—diagnosing is a long process: it took more than half my lifetime for doctors to come up with a diagnosis for me. And that diagnosis is still in flux: overlapping syndromes pop up all the time in lupus patients.

Be a *patient* patient. The best way to deal with this great mimic is to relax and not worry about what the doctors want to call it today: they can call it Fred, for all that it matters. Your lupus will shift and change and develop as you live with it. *Living* with it is what matters.

IN A SENTENCE

Diagnosis is difficult, but living *with* lupus *is your goal.*

"I Feel Like I'm Grieving"

NOW THAT you've had your first day knowing you have lupus, you will find that living with it through the second day, and subsequent days and weeks, is going to be difficult—but not impossible. Living with lupus is often an ongoing process that is very similar to grief and bereavement: some of the cycles of emotions and feelings you will undergo will include anger, denial, the drain of ongoing tests and doctors' visits, as well as learning coping methods and eventual acceptance of how you're going to live with lupus in your daily life.

You feel anger or denial

Both anger and denial are normal for you to feel right now—after all, this is only day two of knowing that you have lupus. You may feel anger about why you have lupus: because no one knows what causes lupus for certain, it's common to feel angry about something over which you feel you have no control and little information. You may feel angry because it took so long to diagnose your disease: lupus, as we discussed in Day One, is very difficult to diagnose and, in fact, may shift (quite a lot, sometimes!) as you continue through your life with it. In fact, you may experience what many lupus patients have: differing diagnoses. You may go to one doctor who says you do have lupus, only to turn to another doctor who says you don't have lupus! No wonder you would feel angry over a situation like that—doctors are supposed to know what they're doing, right? Well, in the case of lupus, because of the conflicting symptoms and overlaps (remember, you can have different symptoms, diseases, and syndromes at the same time), doctors often misdiagnose lupus or miss lupus entirely because they're looking so hard at another disease or syndrome that you already have.

One of my acquaintances with lupus has been diagnosed, undiagnosed, rediagnosed, diagnosed with related lupus conditions, undiagnosed, and rediagnosed more times than she can recall. Every time she sees a new physician, she dreads yet another conflicting diagnosis, or even an entirely new diagnosis of yet another related syndrome. Or a new diagnosis of lupus *again*. One can hardly blame her for feeling angry about doctors.

You may be feeling as if perhaps you don't have lupus after all: didn't that one doctor say you didn't have lupus once upon a time? *Denial* is normal, too. You feel as if after all the backing-and-forthing on your diagnosis that you may not have lupus after all, even though you've now had a definitive diagnosis.

Now that you know it for sure, don't try to keep messing with your mind by telling yourself that you don't have it after all. You've gone through enough with people probably telling you that it's "all in your head," or that you are "exaggerating" your symptoms, or possibly that you don't really have anything wrong with you at all, if you are cycling through flare-ups of symptoms and then are symptom-free. These cycles of being sick then well are *normal* for a lupus patient. Educating yourself, and your friends and family, about these cycles can help stop the denial.

You feel depressed

You may feel *depressed* upon hearing the news that you have lupus. It is a serious disease and many myths are built around it. Depression is normal at this point: it's still only day two.

Depression is actually a commonality between lupus, **chronic fatigue syndrome** (**CFS**), and **fibromyalgia**. Why? These diseases most often affect women, who are often treated by doctors (and, sadly, friends and family) as not having a "serious" disease and/or not having a disease at all, even after diagnosis. Some doctors are taught in medical school that women of a certain age (usually over 30), who are either married but without children, or unmarried, and who have a host of seemingly unconnected complaints are suffering from "difficult woman's syndrome." The women may have legitimate complaints (i.e., lupus), but the "constant complaining" (asking questions, pursuing diagnoses, actively getting involved in her own health treatments) is said to be treated as a psychological sidebar, so to speak; the woman in question is treated as if she is simply a complainer and a nuisance. The problem with this is that lupus is a disease which: (1) affects mostly women, and (2) requires patient responsibility for their ongoing health issues. There's obviously a catch-22 going on here: you're damned if you do, and you're damned if you don't.

This is one reason why many lupus patients get depressed: they're trying to help take care of themselves, but are discouraged from doing so. What to do? I'm afraid my only advice is the hardest one out there: Brave through the discouragement and keep on trying to aid yourself in your own health issues. *You're* the one with lupus, not the doctor. Educate your friends and family as to the difficulties inherent in living with lupus; many of them will try in their turn to support you in your fight against depression.

Other forms of depression are brought on by the obvious: ongoing illness, the fatigue common to lupus and some overlapping syndromes, and chronic pain. Overcoming this sort of depression is harder, and often needs the help of your growing support group of family and friends, as well as the professional help of a health care provider. Social workers, psychologists, and psychiatrists are there to help you with the ongoing needs of feeling depressed about having a chronic, difficult, serious disease. Don't be afraid to seek out such help: it doesn't mean you're "crazy." What it does mean is that you're smart: you have reached out to a professional, knowing that they have the training and knowledge, and perhaps prescriptive abilities, to help you through some of the roughest times you'll have with lupus and depression.

Especially if you have chronic pain that is ongoing and overwhelming, seek out your doctor's advice on what to do about it before you become too depressed to even think of asking for help yourself. Pain is nothing to sneeze at: it can be as debilitating as any other symptom or syndrome associated with lupus, and it can cause depression the fastest.

CONFLICTING DIAGNOSES

Doctors will retest you on a regular basis: this doesn't mean you don't still have lupus. Retesting your blood for certain factors with lupus is very common and will change your diagnosis for the level of severity of your SLE or different overlapping syndromes. All those tests and retests aren't because the doctors necessarily think you don't have lupus: they told you that you do.

However, you may run into a common problem we touched on earlier: conflicting diagnoses. This happens to most people with lupus, sometimes before they get a definitive diagnosis, sometimes after they get their diagnosis, which causes them to rethink and reassess their illness all over again. No wonder you may be feeling angry or denying your diagnosis, or even feeling depressed about it! If two, three, or even four doctors can't agree on your diagnosis, it can be a very frustrating situation.

You are not alone. Almost all lupus patients have this happen. This goes back to what we talked about in Day One—lupus is hard to diagnose and often mimics other diseases and syndromes. It's frustrating; it's depressing; it's infuriating—and it's normal. The best advice I was given by a doctor during my days of multiple, conflicting diagnoses was: Pick the most reliable diagnosis and doctor, and stick with it, for now. For all that doctors are our best-educated and trained people in the health field, they have egos; sometimes those egos bump into each other, often in the *specialty fields,* which is where you're at with a diagnosis of lupus. Sometimes doctors disagree with each other's diagnoses for reasons other than what you may believe—some of the disagreements are because of ongoing research they're involved in personally; some of the disagreements are because of affiliations with particular hospitals or clinics. Some disagreements are because of personal beliefs in the diagnosis of lupus (see sidebar, Day One: the criteria for diagnosing lupus are in dispute).

A trained physician told you that you have lupus; she or he has tests and reliable data to back it up. You feel that the diagnosis is correct. Stand by that doctor, if you believe he or she was right, and go on and *live* with your lupus from there.

Coping methods

Coping with all this anger, denial, depression, and possible ongoing conflicts regarding your diagnosis appears to be a hard task. Well, it is, and it isn't. The biggest help in coping is going to be your support system. We'll talk more about this in Day Three, but suffice it to say that your friends, family, doctor(s), and perhaps new-made friends who also have lupus are going to be valuable support for coping with all these feelings and conflicts.

Don't deny yourself their help. Seek it out—create it, if necessary. Living with lupus can't happen in a vacuum if you expect to cope with all the difficulties inherent in having this disease.

IN A SENTENCE:

> *You may feel anger, denial, and depression from having lupus, but coping with it is possible with help from your support groups.*

learning

Rheumatology

THE SPECIALISTS who deal specifically with lupus are called **rheumatologists**, since lupus is classified along with rheumatoid arthritis and other rheumatological diseases. Unlike rheumatoid arthritis, what lupus does is affect the *connective tissues* rather than the bones themselves, and while swelling, pain, and other effects are found in the joints of lupus patients, by and large lupus does not actually cause lasting damage or destruction of the bones and joints the way arthritis does. Many of the overlapping syndromes, such as **Sjögren's Syndrome**, are also classified with the rheumatological diseases.

What is a rheumatologist & how do I find one?

Rheumatologists are medical doctors (MDs) who have specialized training and studies in the rheumatological diseases. Rheumatologists are the people who can help you with specific questions, tests, and ongoing treatments for lupus. While your regular family physician may be perfectly capable of treating you for most of your lupus symptoms, finding and using a rheumatologist (if you don't already have one from your diagnosis), really is necessary to have the specialized care you will require as a lupus patient.

I have recently run into two instances of women diagnosed with lupus who were not recommended to seek a rheumatologist for treatment—strangely enough, both women go to the same hair salon I attend. Both women were confused, uneducated about their disease, and had primary care physicians who actively discouraged them from seeking out information about lupus. To both of them I offered the same recommendation I offer you here, with the caveat that I am only a *patient,* not a physician myself: *Find a rheumatologist.* And arm yourself by educating yourself about lupus.

Rheumatologists can be found by asking either your family physician for a referral, or through your health insurance plan, which will either have a booklet of specialists on your plan—usually listed by geographical area—or possibly an Internet Web site which will have a searchable database of all physicians, usually divisible by specialty and location. Make sure of your health insurance's requirements for seeing a specialist before setting up appointments and tests with your rheumatologist —many of them require a *referral* by your family physician or primary care physician (PCP, in insurance lingo).

It is critical that you are happy with the rheumatologist that you find—you are going to go through both good and bad times with this physician. It's important that you feel comfortable telling your doctor when you feel a flare-up of lupus symptoms coming on (and yes, you *will* learn how to detect when your symptoms are about to start worsening—more on that in Day Three: Acceptance). You don't want to be in the situation where you are uncomfortable telling your rheumatologist that you're feeling funk, afraid that he or she will chalk up your feelings to "something in your head." Ditto for when you truly are feeling down: you need to be able to tell your doctor when you're feeling down or depressed from the ongoing symptoms or from pain. If you don't feel as if you can confide to your doctor regarding your symptoms, then find another rheumatologist. It's absolutely necessary that you find one who you feel is on your side, supporting you through your life with lupus.

What will the rheumatologist do for me?

Your specialist will be your primary medical support for all issues pertaining to your lupus. On the other hand, if you develop the flu or you fall and break your leg, that's in your family physician's arena. Sometimes medical conditions overlap: flu may develop into pneumonia, which may develop into a **pleural effusion.** In that case, the pleuritis is actually in your rheumatologist's arena, as your immune system is obviously dealing with the unusual: your lupus has caused a normal course of the flu to develop into an inflammation in the lining around your lungs. Your primary care physician will coordinate with your rheumatologist in such situations, making sure you get the best care possible for a patient who just happens to have lupus. This means you also need a PCP who will be comfortable in dealing with a specialist—the same warning as above applies. If you feel uncomfortable with your family physician's dealings with your rheumatologist, it's time to look at a new family doctor. Everyone is going to have to play together nicely in this sandbox.

Your rheumatologist will conduct ongoing tests for your lupus symptoms, for overlapping syndromes if they develop, and for your entire system, as it is related to the various medications you will be placed on. Lupus patients have to have several body systems monitored on an ongoing basis, usually every six months, both because they can be affected by the lupus itself and by the medicines most patients take. Your rheumatologist will also conduct all the preliminary tests for lupus every so often, to check for levels in your blood, symptoms of your skin, organs, connective tissues, and other body functions, to see how you are doing. Often your rheumatologist can spot an upcoming flare of symptoms this way, even before you start feeling it yourself.

Preliminary lupus testing

You may have been diagnosed with lupus without the full battery of tests, or you may have already had all these done. Either way, you will probably have some if not all of these done over again on an occasional basis by your rheumatologist, just to see how you're faring.

BLOOD TESTS

- ○ ANA
- ○ C Reactive Protein
- ○ sedimentation rate
- ○ serum protein electrophoresis
- ○ standard CBC panel (complete blood count)
- ○ complement components (such as complement C3 and C4)
- ○ autoantibodies (such as anti-DNA, anti-Ro/SS-A, anti-RNP, or anti-SM)
- ○ liver and kidney functions (#AST, ALT, BUN, creatinine)
- ○ serum albumin

OTHER TESTS

Some other tests include listening to the lungs for a *pleural rub,* which is the sound made when breathing deeply that indicates an inflammation in the pleural lining surrounding the lungs. Many lupus patients suffer from pleurisy (inflammation) and pleuritis (inflammation with a liquid effusion) and frequent pneumonia, in season, since the pleural lining is a rather large section of connective tissue in the body and is related to immune system regulation.

Your doctor will probably test your wrists, elbows, knees, and ankles for movement, looking for arthritis symptoms, as both osteo- and rheumatoid arthritis are not uncommon for those with lupus. He or she will ask if you are losing hair (unrelated to pattern hair loss in both men and women), if you have mouth sores, if you have unusually dry eyes or mouth, or if you have any rashes. She may also ask if you are finding yourself sensitive to sunlight. Any of these questions sound familiar? They were listed in the previous chapter in the sidebar of standard diagnosis for lupus. Your doctor is looking for the development of new symptoms, as lupus is not a static disease but an ongoing process. You will develop some new syndromes and symptoms, and lose others, as you move on with the disease throughout your life.

Expect your doctor to continue asking these questions, over and over again, every year or every six months. He is not being redundant—he's being a good rheumatologist, and he's being a thorough specialist by seeking out changes in your disease by going down the list of preliminary diagnosis each time you see him for a checkup.

Ongoing tests

The ongoing tests, aside from repetition of the preliminary tests we discussed above, will vary depending on your particular symptoms and your medications.

Most lupus patients take a form of nonsteroidal anti-inflammatory (NSAID), such as Celebrex or Vioxx. These drugs affect the COX-2 enzymes in the body, reducing inflammation caused by the disease. Unfortunately, they also can have the side effect of placing both your stomach and kidneys under stress. Your stomach may develop ulcers—these can be tested for through a variety of means, most particularly an upper-GI scan using barium in a "milkshake," which you swallow (they can flavor it—it really isn't as awful as it sounds), and a live X-ray picture then follows it down your throat and into your stomach, showing where any abrasions or erosions are going on.

Any kidney damage can be discovered early on by a blood test which looks for reduced kidney function before it can become a serious problem for the patient. Since each person taking NSAIDs reacts in a different way to them, changing brands can clear up problems as well as cause the particular NSAID to work more or less efficiently for you. A study done at Brigham Young University in 2002, reported in *Science*

News (Sept. 21, 2002, Vol. 162, No. 12), looks into this very subject, regarding NSAIDs and individual reactions to the drugs' interactions with the COX-2 enzymes responsible for inflammation. The study actually is about the COX-3 inhibitor, **acetaminophen**, and how it can interact with COX-1 and COX-2. One result was the realization that different nonsteroidal anti-inflammatories work differently for different people, perhaps showing that the COX enzymes may be structured differently in each person. The study's results goes a long way to explain why one person can take Celebrex and have it work like a charm for arthritis and other inflammatory symptoms, while for another person it does little good at all.

Your rheumatologist may also test on an ongoing basis for various overlapping conditions that he or she may think you will develop, such as Raynaud's Syndrome, Sjögren's Syndrome, or fibromyalgia. She may not think you actually have one of these syndromes in addition to your systemic lupus, but she may think that, given the range and cluster of symptoms you already have (which are individual for each lupus patient), you may be a candidate in the future for one or more of these syndromes, and she will want to catch it sooner rather than later. More on what these syndromes do, and how tests are conducted for them, will be discussed during both Day Six and Month Three.

IN A SENTENCE:

> *Finding a good rheumatologist, who will support you with ongoing care and testing, is very important in helping to cope with lupus.*

living

Accepting
Your Lupus

COMING TO an acceptance of your life with lupus will
include not only your own experience of coping with the disease in your life, but also telling your family and friends
about how they can become part of your support mecha-
nism, recognizing an oncoming flare of lupus before it over-
whelms you, and educating yourself about the importance of
diet, rest, and exercise, all taken in their measure. You will
also need to integrate some pain management techniques
into your lifestyle, for those times when flares of symptoms
are unavoidable. All of these are necessary in order to continue accepting that lupus is now part of your life—a man-
ageable part of your life.

Friends and Family

Oftentimes your family and friends have already become
part of a support network for you while you have been sick
and seeking a diagnosis. Sometimes, however, you will have

friends and family who have been disbelieving that your disease was "serious," or that you even had one, passing it off instead as something that was "all in your head," since you have had so many varying symptoms that have come and gone, leaving the people around you feeling perplexed and perhaps even angry. Does this reaction sound familiar? You may have felt that way yourself at one point while you were still undiagnosed, and again right after diagnosis, uncertain how to cope with the anger and denial inherent in finding out you have lupus.

You may find yourself in the position of having to educate your family and friends about your disease. Take the opportunity to talk to them about lupus—gift them with a copy of this book. The more they know about lupus, the better positioned they will be to help you when you do get sick during a flare-up. It's important for them to *know* that you have a serious, but not necessarily fatal, disease, and that they can help you by their knowledge. They will know that you will need to change certain aspects of your lifestyle, make compromises, and even perhaps adjust your work schedule. Your family and friends may even be in a position to help you with all of this.

This support network will become invaluable to you throughout your life. People who know you, and understand how lupus is affecting your life, will be able to support you in your decisions regarding your healthcare and your lifestyle changes necessary to maintain a healthy mind and body. Having people on your side is especially helpful when you start to slide into the dumps when you undergo a flare—they can remind you of the positive aspects of living with lupus and help you with what you need to do to come out the other side of a flare-up. You will inevitably encounter people who will never understand what you're undergoing; turn to your support network at these times. This is when they can be of the greatest help.

Am I getting a flare?

Flares are what doctors refer to when your lupus becomes active. Flares can be anything from an increase in existing symptoms to the development of new ones. Flares are often preceded by a slow or subtle change in your daily lupus symptoms—perhaps you may start becoming more easily tired than usual, or you may start feeling as if you're coming down with the flu, but it never develops into a real flu.

Flares are a natural part of lupus, and they're what your new support structure of friends and family are going to help you through. Knowing your particular signs of an oncoming flare is important for your support people to recognize, as you may not be in a position to recognize them yourself. They also need to recognize when you're in need of support and not asking for it—don't deny them the pleasure of helping you out!

Having flares, then going into remission (periods of little or no illness caused directly by the lupus) is both normal and frustrating. Remember that acceptance of the cycle of flares as part of your life is important for both you and your support network.

Pain management

Pain is going to become part of your life with lupus, whether it's pain from an overlapping condition such as fibromyalgia or from a flare-up of pleurisy or from the discomfort of digestive problems caused by inflammation. Knowing and understanding, and *accepting*, your pain is part of a life with lupus.

Don't be afraid to tell your support network—which includes your family physician and rheumatologist—that you are in pain. They can't help you with pain management if you don't let them. Also, don't be afraid to listen to the advice of others who think you might be in pain, even if you don't realize it yourself. Pain can manifest itself in insidious ways: I've often been in a great deal of pain from a flare, unaware of it until my husband tells me, "Nancy, you're in pain. Go lie down now." My shouted response is inevitably cut short when I realize that I've been grousing about nitpicking details of something trivial for hours and am really in pain instead. I go lie down, grateful for such a supportive spouse.

Pain can be managed in many ways, including the use of medications (not all of which make you groggy—there are many on the market now that do wonders without the "old" side effects), exercise, **biofeedback**, meditation, and talk therapy. If you feel you are encountering pain levels that interfere with your sleep or with your ability to progress normally through a day, talk to your doctors about the possibility of using a pain management center for diagnosis and treatment of your pain. Most middle- to large-sized hospitals have a pain management center associated with them, even in some remote areas of the country.

Both rest & exercise are important

Although this sounds contradictory, for lupus patients both rest *and* exercise are important. Why both? Because those of us with lupus have different symptoms, and different needs for body movement at different times during flares and remissions.

Adequate sleep is extremely important for those with lupus because a great deal of the body's immune system is regulated by sleep. Ever hear as a kid that you "can't grow if you don't sleep"? It's been proven true by medical studies that the human growth hormone, occurring naturally in the body, is suppressed if children don't get enough sleep. This same hormone contributes to the healthy lives of adults, including adults with lupus. Ever tried to get over a bad flu on not enough sleep? Bet you just couldn't shake that bug—that's because the immune system relies on sleep, the "downtime" of the body, to make correct repairs. Your immune system is already confused because of lupus—let's not confuse it further by depriving it of sleep.

Exercise is equally important to keep your immune system healthy, stimulating the correct pathways of healing and cellular growth. "But I'm in pain," you may counter. There are limits to some types of exercise certain lupus patients may be capable of performing, depending on their symptoms and other conditions carried with the lupus. You may have arthritis that precludes you from lifting weights in a certain manner—but did you know that doing weight-bearing exercise only three times a week for twenty minutes (studies disagree on the exact amount, but this is the average) can help prevent bone loss through osteoporosis? If you are a woman approaching menopause, osteoporosis may be in your future soon—men aren't off the hook, either, as they lose bone mass as they age, as well. And weight-bearing exercise, such as lifting low-weight hand weights, can help prevent further damage from osteoarthritis and the pain from muscle-affected syndromes such as fibromyalgia.

Nonweight-bearing exercise can be of great benefit as well, particularly if it includes stretching. Yoga and Pilates are both disciplines that should be investigated by people with lupus who are in pain from doing other types of exercise.

Working through moderate pain by doing exercise stimulates the release of endorphins from the brain, which make us literally feel good, too. A good workout of twenty minutes of cardiovascular exercise, such as using a recumbent bicycle or walking at a good clip, can make you feel better than all the pain relievers in the world. Doing this at least three times a week has helped me immensely—buying a membership to a local gym, and finding a trainer who has some knowledge of lupus herself, has been a godsend for my own life with lupus.

Always—always, *always!*—check with your doctors before beginning a new exercise regime. He or she will want to check your resting pulse, cardiac and pulmonary functions, and give you guidelines to gain the most from any exercise that you do. Having lupus means special care must be taken to not radically change anything affecting your body without talking to your doctor first. But don't forget to ask—don't let this be an excuse to forget about exercise altogether. Sitting on the couch and eating BonBons isn't the answer to life with lupus, either.

DIET & NUTRITION

Weight gain or loss is equally important in the life of a person with lupus. Often a diagnosis of lupus will come after someone rapidly loses weight due to a particular symptom or period of illness. Weight gain can come from any number of avenues, most particularly medications such as **Prednisone** or **Medrol** (nonanabolic **corticosteroids**, which reduce inflammation) or NSAIDs (nonsteroidal anti-inflammatories), or lack of exercise because of a protracted illness or chronic pain.

There is a great deal of debate about the role of nutrition in the life of a person with lupus. No one doubts that proper nutrition following standard FDA guidelines is paramount: eating the correct proportions of protein, carbohydrates, and fat—all in their correct amounts—is necessary for anyone's health. But beyond that, no one seems to be able to agree. Some people claim that higher protein diets (such as the one used for the American Diabetes Association) are better for lupus; some say higher carbohydrate diets (the old "pyramid" diet, which is still the FDA's standard) is better. Some say that additives and processed food can trigger flares in lupus patients, and may even contribute to the development of lupus in people who already have a predisposition to getting it. Others say that particular vitamins, minerals, or other dietary supplements aid in keeping lupus flares from occurring, or getting flares to go away.

I can't speak definitively to this issue other than to encourage you to do your own research on this matter, aided by the appendix in the back of this book of further reading materials, and speak with your doctors about it. I, personally, have made two changes to my life which *appear* to help my lupus flares.

First, I have tried to stay away from foods that are highly processed and full of additives, particularly foods that are sprayed with pesticides or treated with hormones, such as fresh vegetables, beef and chicken, and milk. In fact, one of my allergies turned out to be milk—something that an ER doctor figured out, after the particular symptom of severe gastric distress stumped everyone, including my rheumatologist of the time—cutting it out of my diet cleared up a lot. Being checked for food allergies isn't necessarily a bad idea, since lupus patients seem to have a large amount of anecdotal testimony attributing certain symptoms to food allergies, including the "lupus headache," which can often be helped by eliminating migraine-causing foods from the diet.

Because lupus is a disease affecting the immune system, and because we know that certain hormones and additives affect the immune system's natural rhythms, I figured it would be best to know *exactly* what was in my food. Mystery meat was fine while I was eating at the college cafeteria, but no longer. Through studies done, particularly in Boston in the 1980s, we also know that certain chemicals appear to trigger the onset of lupus, particularly in women. Again, I figured that cutting chemicals as far out of my life as possible, especially in the foods that I eat, would be better than not knowing what was going into my already-confused body.

Second, I have been taking vitamin B-family multivitamins ever since seeing the first doctor to suggest lupus to me as a diagnosis. He had been reading a number of studies that showed a link between taking vitamin B complex family and preventing, or at least calming, the flare-up of lupus symptoms in certain women. Surely it couldn't hurt, I thought—after all, I should be taking them as part of a premenstrual formula anyway. So I started on a women's formula multivitamin with the prescribed doses of vitamin B complex he recommended and found relief from a number of symptoms of lupus flares. And I found when I didn't take my vitamins for a number of months, I got those same symptoms back again.

Again, this is only the anecdotal evidence of one person, though there have been a number of medical studies done on both issues I note above. I am not prescribing that you follow what I've done. I can tell you that *no one* recommends a high-protein diet that could put stress on kidney function, since lupus patients already have stresses on their kidneys without adding more. What I do recommend is that you set up a time to either talk with your doctor, or a referred nutritionist who is trained about lupus, and set up some guidelines for both your daily diet needs—whether or not you need to gain or lose weight—and to discuss issues such as supplements and food content/preparation.

IN A SENTENCE:

> *In order to fully accept your life with lupus, you must learn more about it and take actions through pain management and lifestyle management.*

learning

Starting to Learn More About Lupus

NOW YOU'RE starting to learn more about this disease called lupus. You've learned the basics about what lupus is and what it can do. Now you can start to do some more in-depth research on what lupus will mean in your life, how to find reliable information about lupus and related diseases and syndromes, and where to find help and support for your life with lupus.

Researching lupus on the Internet

If you're like me, one of the first things you did on hearing that you have lupus was to rush home to your computer, fire up the modem, and go onto the Internet. The Net has become our own personal research library, in many ways, over the last five to ten years. Since the introduction of the World Wide Web, finding information on the Net has become even easier.

But it's also easier to find *too much* information, and information that's not necessarily reliable. I want to take a minute here, not to give you a bunch of Web site links, but to talk about how do to reliable research on the Net. We'll get to the links later—check out the appendix, where I list both places to read about lupus and organizations to help you with support for lupus.

NOT EVERYTHING YOU READ ON THE NET IS TRUE

I know this may be blaringly obvious to some people, but I want to repeat this again: *Not everything you read on the Net is necessarily true.* You need to learn who has written the material; you need to learn if it comes from a credible and known source or institution; you need to dig deeper than the "front page." Some Web sites about lupus are personal testimonials. These can be great as far as they go, particularly if you are looking for stories to let you know that you "aren't the only one." But they're also not a recipe for how to then conduct proper nutrition *for you,* what medications to take *for you,* or what symptoms indicate illnesses or syndromes *you* have. Only your doctor can give you that information. Getting information from Mary Sue Whipple's personal Web site may be a great beginning to give you some new ideas, but never, *ever* go off and change your diet or try a new herbal supplement or even try some radical new exercise regime based on her Web site. Again, only you and your doctor can make those determinations. What worked for her, almost guaranteed, won't necessarily work for you. Besides, are you sure she actually got the name of that herbal supplement right? You could take something that will interfere with a medication you're on—and that can lead to disastrous results.

LOOK FOR PRIMARY SOURCES OF INFORMATION

What is a primary source of information? Not the Web site of a testimonial for a commercial product that refers to the abstract of a study done in 1999 by Ubo Research Group. What you want to look for is the study *itself.* If the paper isn't available in full-text format on the Net, check and see if you can buy a copy of the article from a magazine that published the study. Check with resources such as your local librarian to see if the article is in a magazine that they carry, or can order through interlibrary loan. If the study is too technical for you, consider broadening your search for information to reliable sources of primary information that abstract and/or abridge them for the consumer or nonprofessional.

RELIABLE SOURCES OF INFORMATION

Check out reliable, professional sources of information about lupus, not all of which are situated at for-professionals-only medical Web sites. Take heed of the advice above: make sure these sites are part of accredited associations or medical groups that carry primary sources of information about lupus, not just secondary information or testimonials.

WebMD (www.webmd.com) offers abstracts and reprints of medical papers, even on their consumer side of the Web site. The same goes for other medical sites to which consumers can get access, even if they also have access for medical professionals. A short list of such Web sites is included in the appendix of Suggested Reading.

Don't forget to look at the resources available online from the national and international associations for various syndromes associated with lupus and, of course, lupus itself. One of the best such sources is the Lupus Foundation of America, which keeps full-text versions of all their educational materials and pamphlets online (www.lupus.org). Almost all syndromes that show up in overlapping cases of lupus have at least one site of their own, if not more (fibromyalgia has about five different associations in North America alone).

The Lupus Foundation of America

This nonprofit foundation is one of the best sources of information about lupus and ongoing research in the field. You can reach their Web site at: www.lupus.org, or write to them for a list of their educational materials and pamphlets at:

Lupus Foundation of America, Inc.
1300 Piccard Drive, Suite 200
Rockville, MD 20850-4303
Phone: (301) 670-9292 9 AM–5 PM (ET) Monday–Friday
Fax: (301) 670-9486
1-800-558-0121 (Information request line)
1-800-558-0231 (Para información en Español)

You can subscribe to their newsletter, *Lupus News,* for $25 a year within the U.S. (international subscriptions are available). From their site, you can also find information about local chapters of the LFA, most of which also have their own newsletters and informative packets or pamphlets.

Finding local support

Local support groups can be found outside the Lupus Foundation of America sanctioned chapters. Many hospitals and clinics have lupus support groups that meet monthly, giving you the option of something that may be closer than the LFA chapter meeting for your state or region. Ask your rheumatologist if he or she knows of a local support group—you may be surprised to find out that there's one that meets not only in your closest town or city, but may even have members whom you already know.

Local groups can be of great help when you're going through a tough time with finding a new doctor or specialist, if your friends or family aren't as supportive as you wish they were, or if you are going through the inevitable questions of "am I the only one who ? . . ." Sometimes only other people who have lupus can help people with lupus—you can support each other, cry with each other, help each other find answers to medical questions, and even laugh with each other (who better to laugh with over a "lupus mask" story?). When family gets you down, or you just need to talk to people you *know* understand what you're going through, try a local group. These groups are usually moderated by a medical professional, social worker, or other person trained in group dynamics, which can help alleviate any of the fears of "but what if the group gets out of hand?"

The hardest part is getting to a group when you are in the middle of a flare or an illness caused by the lupus. When that happens, you often need to talk to your peers the most, but you aren't physically capable of going out to a meeting. When this happens, luckily there is another option these days: the Internet.

Online support groups

From the early days of CompuServe, AOL, and GEnie dialup Internet accounts of the 1980s, through the beginning of the Web and now into the age of broadband Internet access, support groups for people with illnesses such as lupus have been at the forefront of online community development. After all, what better way to use remote communications than by using it to bring people together who need support but are unable to travel to meet in groups?

I would issue the same sort of warnings about online support groups for lupus that I would for "real world" groups:

- Make sure the group meets or communicates regularly.
- Make sure the group has a moderator(s) who has some training in group dynamics or a professional medical background.
- Make sure everyone in the group is there for the purpose of support, not self-aggrandizement or research (unless you *know and want* to join a research group, in which case make absolutely sure it is part of a legitimate study and privacy issues are addressed in writing).

Unlike groups that meet in a physical environment, online support groups have the added benefit that they can often be instant support for you at any time of day or night.

There are three basic types of online communities:

○ live chat based
○ bulletin-board based
○ e-mail based

Any one of these three can be used for online support groups, but they are often combined, so you can have live/instant conversation and feedback from people who have lupus, just like you, and bulletin boards or e-mail lists that provide an ongoing *text* community that has an archival history of discussions and information shared between its members.

I always look for a combination community when I'm looking at a new online support group. The group which I first joined when diagnosed with lupus, and to which I still belong and rely upon for support, is a small community of writers and editors who are united by their work in science fiction. We have a mailing list plus an Internet Relay Chat (IRC) chat system we use for live talking, mostly in the evenings (many people with lupus suffer from insomnia—not surprising, our online "chat room" is often called "Insomniacs"). Belonging to this group helped me especially in the early days of diagnosis, but more so when I was laid up with hemorrhagic pneumonia and again with a blood clot in my leg, both of which prevented me from moving very far from my bed or desk.

Having a support group outside my family—who assuredly were tired of answering what to them were unanswerable questions, such as, "Does anybody else with lupus have X happen to them?" or "How come Y is happening to me right now?"—was invaluable during those flares. Only other "lupoids" were of help to me during some of those long nights.

IN A SENTENCE:

> *Your friends and family, as well as local and online lupus support groups, can aid you in learning more about lupus and attaining positive lifestyle management.*

Stress

STRESS IS a big factor in your life with lupus—both experiencing stress and learning how to manage the stress. Lupus is a disease that, because of its nature of literally flaring up and then receding, causes stress because you never know when you may suddenly come down sick. It's rather like standing in a field and never knowing when lightning will strike out of an open, blue sky. No wonder people with lupus feel stressed! Add to that people you meet, or possibly even friends or family, who put stress on you because they don't understand the nature of your disease and expect you to act "normally," and you have a recipe for a stressful life.

What to do about it? Lowering stress can be handled in many ways—let's look at a few of them and then talk about what you can do to help *others* help *you* reduce pressures in your life. The big lesson to learn here is: *The less stress in your life, the more likelihood of reducing the number of lupus flares you will experience.* Flares are directly influenced by stress. Pressures on your life put pressure on the way your body handles stress, which in turn is handled by the immune system's response. The immune system in a person with lupus is already confused—by putting stress on the system, you are confusing it even more, causing the possibility of more flares.

Lower your stress levels

Early on, I was advised by many people, and by reading many articles on lupus, to reduce the stress in my life in order to help manage the disease. This advice isn't bad for anyone, but is critical for the lupus patient. Anecdotal evidence from most people with lupus shows that stress in their lives heralds an oncoming flare by only a few weeks or even days. Avoiding that stress in the first place can keep the dreaded flares at bay to a great extent.

It isn't easy to change your life, especially if you've been living "in the fast lane" both for work and play. Take a look at what you do during a normal day and see how you can cut out stressful encounters and experiences without diminishing what you feel is the quality of your lifestyle. Remember, stress can sometimes hide behind a normally enjoyable event or activity. You may love boating, but the act of going to the marina, launching the boat, spending the day out on the water, coming back to harbor, and driving home again may stress your body, thus putting you at greater risk for a flare. When we define stress here, we don't necessarily mean things that only make you *unhappy*; we mean anything that causes a strain on your system or makes you feel tired from the activity or event.

Make a diary of your activities and their stress levels—see the box on the next page and copy it. Fill it out and see what patterns emerge. What activity is making you stressful? What activity is making you relaxed?

It's possible that your life has already changed significantly long before you were diagnosed definitively with lupus—most lupus patients have undergone a long string of illnesses and symptoms that led up to their diagnosis. You may feel you've already lost whatever quality of lifestyle you had in "the before-time" (before lupus). In this case, you need to look at how you can regain a feeling of quality in your life by

Daily Stress Diary

TIME	ACTIVITY What, where, with whom	STRESS LEVEL Very stressful, Somewhat stressful, Not very stressful, Relaxing
7am		
8am		
9am		
10am		
11am		
Noon		
1pm		
2pm		
3pm		
4pm		
5pm		
6pm		
7pm		
8pm		
9pm		
10pm		
11pm		

adding back in activities that cause little or no stress but can "get the job done" in spite of your disease.

Lowering stress at work

Lowering stress levels at work can possibly be the trickiest part of changing your lifestyle as a person with lupus. Some people have very little control over their work environment and are in positions where they can't change how much stress is placed on them by those higher up or outside their work group. This is going to sound trite, but there really are only four options when you have little control over stress in your workplace:

1. Talk to those in charge and see how you can create a less stressful work environment.
2. Ask to be placed on flex-time (flexible hours) or possibly go on part-time work.
3. Ask to be placed as a consultant to work remotely at home, if this is possible in your profession and workplace.
4. Consider changing jobs.

Possibilities exist in many jobs—in technology fields, especially—for flex-time and changes in the work environment itself. While doing consultancy work for a dot-com two years ago, I spoke ahead of time to my boss before going down to Texas for a week of in-house work, and asked for the following conditions:

○ A sofa or other place available for a short nap in the afternoon
○ A chair/desk setup that allowed me to keep my feet elevated (I have typical blood clotting problems found in some lupus patients)
○ The ability to come in later and leave later at night (for me, at least, lupus has made me a seriously *non*-morning-person)

No one had any problem with these conditions, though I think many of my colleagues wished they could also take a nap in the afternoon! After explaining how lupus works for me, and armed with the knowledge that reducing stress would allow me to work longer and produce better results for the company, I was supported in my needs and we had a lot of fun in the process.

Reducing your income by going to part-time hours, or even changing your career entirely, may be an inevitable outcome of stress reduction for many people. A good friend from my online support community, Wolfbytes, writes:

> My life has changed considerably: I'm no longer able to hold down the high-powered career that once fueled my income because I quite simply cannot work every day. I've moved from my nine-room Victorian into a four-room rental; from a new, highway-safe car every few years to a twenty-year-old, "locally depend-able" vehicle. I've watched two careers slide into the realms of impossible.
>
> And still I hold onto the thought, even knowing how futile it is, that one day I'll wake up, the losses of the past fourteen years will be restored, and *I'll* be restored to health and my prior status. This is not unique to me; I've talked to many chronically ill people who feel, hope, pray, delude themselves for and with the same thoughts. And yet, I have learned to live with it. (Modean Moon, via e-mail, 9/23/02: used with permission)

The hard part is coming to terms with this one fact: *Your life is not going to be like it was before.* There's no way around that: you have lupus, and it changes your life, whether you want it to or not. Having a measure of control over those changes, by making decisions yourself and changing your workplace habits or working life before they're forcibly changed for you, can help ease you into this new life with lupus. There will be a measure of compromise: if you decide to go to part-time work, you're going to see a drop in income. Some of your changes are going to be difficult ones to make.

Many people looking to reduce stress induced by work look toward career changes such as consultancy work (though this brings its own stress with it, especially if the person involved has problems with self-motivation), freelance work, home-based businesses, and even writing. This is often where your lupus support group can be of help: talk to them about how they have reduced stress at work, how they've changed careers or directions for work. You may end up getting some very good advice, indeed, from people who do understand your situation.

Reducing stress at home

Stress at home can be just as difficult as stress at work, especially for women. Most women are trying to juggle career, husband, children, and home—and once lupus or another chronic disease hits, they're left feeling as if they are overwhelmed by just *one* of those aspects of their life, never mind all four!

How can you deal with the stress you have at home? First of all, start looking at that diary of daily activity and see where the stress comes up in your life. Are you stressed out because you have to do the dishes every morning before leaving for work? Can someone else start doing the dishes for you? Can your family afford a dishwasher? (Put in the context of you spending a week in bed with a flare, every month or so, that dishwasher may seem like good economics.)

Stress doesn't have to feel overwhelming. Take it one step at a time. Take all those little stresses from your daily diary and go through them sequentially:

1. Identify the stress factor.
2. Prioritize how important the activity is in your life.
3. Identify which activities can be fulfilled without your involvement or with reduced involvement.
4. Identify ways in which those activities can be handled by others and by whom—and don't be afraid to assign them out!

Home can be just as difficult as work inasfar as people around you, including your family, need to be educated as to what lupus is and how stress will affect you. It's sometimes hard for others, especially our family, to accept that we have lupus: after all, most days you won't "look" as if you're "sick." Preventing getting sick, by reducing stress, will be the key; talk to your family—hold a family meeting as often as you

IF YOU have a cat, and a cat litter box, you should beware of **toxoplasmosis**—an illness caused by a sporozoan that can flourish in cat feces (and therefore in the litter box). This illness is more easily transmitted to those who have compromised or overactive immune systems, such as those with lupus. Because you are more susceptible to toxoplasmosis, you may want to see if your spouse or children can help with the cat litter cleaning chores. If you can't convince someone to help you out, be sure to wear disposable gloves when cleaning the box. You can buy boxes of medical gloves (both latex and latex-free) at any standard pharmacy/drugstore. And don't forget to dispose of the gloves in a safe manner—they can also carry the sporozoan after you handle the dirty cat litter!

need to—and tell them how stress can and does affect how sick or well you'll be with lupus.

Your family loves you, and armed with enough information on how to keep you well, they will be your best defense against flares of your disease. But remember this will work only *if* they know how to help you. You need to keep the lines of communication open and tell them how to help—your spouse and children aren't mind readers. With time, unfortunately enough, they'll start to recognize the signs of an oncoming flare, perhaps even before you. Listen to them, and learn from them, as well as teach them how to help you.

Use your support group

Don't forget to use your support group! I know I may sound like a broken record by now, but I know that many people are like myself: once you learn enough about a subject, you feel you can go off on your own and deal with it alone. After all, you're smart enough to figure out anything that may come up now, right?

Unfortunately, with a chronic illness, it isn't the same as learning a new craft or a new subject from a textbook. There's a lot you can learn from reading and going to lectures, but nothing will replace the support you can receive from a group of like-minded people who are dealing with the same issues as yourself.

Use your support group to help lower stress. Whether your support group meets in person or over the Internet, use your support group to help lower your stress by using them as a sounding board, as a "bitch" session, or just simply as a place to ask questions. You're all there to help each other; chances are, others have either gone through or are going through the same things you are—at work, at home, with friends, with family.

Using the group to reduce stress by simply complaining about your latest ache or pain is a great way to help each other, too. We know what it's like, and we know the fear that our complaints will fall on ears that have heard us complain one too many times. But a group of people *with* lupus understands that kvetching about that stupid butterfly rash, or swollen ankles, or arthritis suddenly flaring up, is something that helps us reduce our stress by getting it out and heard by knowing ears. On the other side of the fence, when a member of your group complains to you about her latest bout of migraines, sometimes the best thing you can do is reciprocate by just plain *listening*.

Don't be afraid to complain to your group to help lower your stress, and don't be afraid to listen to their complaints in turn. That's what support is all about.

IN A SENTENCE:

> *Lowering your stress levels is key to maintaining a healthy life with lupus.*

learning

Frequently Asked Questions about Living with Lupus

LUPUS CAN be a confusing disease, as you've probably figured out by now. There are so many different ways it can affect the body, the mind, and our lives; add all that to the fact that lupus affects each person differently, and you have a recipe for instant stress.

Let's lower your stress a little by answering some frequently asked questions about living with lupus.

I've just been told I have lupus. Am I going to die?

Lupus is a serious disease, but it is not necessarily a fatal disease. Most people who develop lupus end up living a full lifetime. I know how scary the diagnosis can be, but having severe lupus *does not mean you will necessarily die of it.* By taking care of yourself, listening to your doctor, listening to your own body, and taking the medicines you are prescribed, you should live a full life. Remember, you can *live* with lupus!

Throughout this book we will explore various ways in which you can help reduce lupus flares, thus increasing your chances of living a life with lupus primarily in remission. The more you are in remission, the greater your chances to live a long life with fewer complications and secondary conditions that can be caused by lupus.

I've been diagnosed with "severe" lupus. What does that mean?

Severe lupus simply means your lupus can act more "severely," or harshly, on your body than some other people's lupus. It does mean that you'll need to listen to your doctor's advice and pay particular attention to learning your body's signals for an oncoming flare. You need to monitor your stress levels carefully, so you don't get flares that can then turn into severe illness (see the "Living" section of this chapter for a chart to track your stress levels).

Overlapping conditions as well as illnesses from lupus—such as pneumonia, pleurisy, pericarditis, etc.—are what endanger lupus patients. We will take a look at a number of these conditions in the following chapters of this book, especially Months Two through Nine.

I've been prescribed to take "steroids" for my lupus. Does this mean I'm going to look like a weight builder and get all crazy?

The type of drug prescribed for lupus that are referred to as "steroids" are corticosteroids—usually the brand names Prednisone or Medrol. These are not the same as metabolic steroids, which have become infamous for their illegal use by athletes. Unlike metabolic steroids, what corticosteroids do is regulate your body's inflammation response. Lupus causes inflammation because your body is trying to "attack" other perfectly good parts of your body—corticosteroids can suppress that response. Unfortunately, the side effects of drugs like Prednisone don't buff you up like a weightlifter; in fact, they often cause weight gain that is difficult to lose once you have it. We'll discuss the specific effects in Week Two: Learning. Luckily, courses of corticosteroids are usually short-lived.

I used to be able to hold down three courses in college, work several part-time jobs, and do research—all at the same time. Now I feel like I'm lucky to remember my own telephone number. I'm terrified I'm losing my mind. What's happening to me? Is it the lupus?

Lupus often causes what, for lack of a better term, is usually called "brain fog." Now that you've heard me use that term, you're probably nodding your head and thinking, "Yes! That's just what it's like: being in a fog." *You aren't losing your mind.* The fog will come and go, usually determined by your stress levels and also by any ongoing or upcoming flare. No one really knows what causes this condition, but it may be related to your autoimmune responses to a flare and inflammation levels in your body. No matter what causes the "fog" clinically, what's important to *you* is learning how to cope with it while it's happening. We'll look more at that in Week Four.

I'm bone-tired all the time, but I feel as if I should be able to do as much as before I was diagnosed with lupus. Some days I'm so tired, no one can wake me up, and I fall asleep in the middle of conversations. People are telling me to just "buck up" and "get on with my life," but I'm so very tired. What's up with all that?

What you're experiencing isn't just "being tired"; you have clinical fatigue. You need to learn to pace yourself and listen to your body: if you're experiencing fatigue at those levels, you need to talk to your PCP or rheumatologist and figure out if there are medications or other techniques to help you through your fatigue periods. If the fatigue doesn't let up, you may have what's called Chronic Fatigue Syndrome (CFS), which sometimes accompanies lupus and other autoimmune diseases. We'll discuss CFS in more detail in Day Seven. For now, know that those of us with clinical fatigue are with you—I suffer from it, and I know full well that when people tell me to "just buck up," I want to shout back at them, "You don't know what it's like! I'm not being lazy!" Try to educate the people around you (hand them this book, for instance) so they can support you rather than cause more stress—and therefore more fatigue.

Why is lupus called "lupus"?

Lupus comes from the Latin form of the word for *wolf*. Many people with lupus develop the malar rash or "lupus mask" that looked like a bite from a wolf to early doctors who identified lupus as a disease. They named the disease after this masking effect. (Personally, I end up looking more like a raccoon, but I rather like the idea of the disease being named after wolves than after raccoons!)

Can I have children?

Early on, female lupus patients were discouraged from having children for fear that it would stress their bodies to the point of kidney failure or worse. As late as the 1980s, this was still often the case with certain doctors' advice. Nowadays, however, doctors realize that with proper prenatal attention to the pregnant woman, stress levels on the body can be maintained to the point where having a baby won't cause any more outrageous flare-ups of lupus than usual. Talk to your doctor and rheumatologist about the idea of pregnancy if you would like to consider having children—there's little reason to think they will discourage you from it.

This does, however, also bring up the topic of passing along possible lupus genetic tendencies in any children you might have. The latest research, as of May 2003, shows that there is probably a genetic *tendency* toward lupus, but there's no way to tell if any one person with that tendency will actually develop the disease. All manner of things have to happen to cause the gene—found on chromosome 1—to "break," causing lupus to surface. The answer is we simply don't know enough yet to say whether or not you can really pass lupus on to children; in the end it is your decision, formed with information from research and your doctor.

We will explore this further in Month Ten.

What causes lupus?

As discussed in Day One: Learning, we don't really know what causes lupus, but we do know this much: (1) it is a complex genetic disease, meaning some people will have a predisposition to develop it, (2) only 10% of those people with the genetic marker in their family develop the disease, (3) more women than men develop lupus, and (4) lupus is sometimes triggered by drug exposure, light sensitivity exposure, and other environmental factors. The Lupus Foundation of America and other like organizations around the world are working on finding out just what causes lupus. Hopefully, in our lifetimes, the cause(s) of lupus will be found, which will be a major step forward in finding a way to either cure or at least predict lupus behavior.

IN A SENTENCE:

> *Despite the hard questions about what lupus is and how it affects the body, lupus is a disease that can be lived with and a full lifespan can be anticipated.*

DAY **5**

living

Doctors
and Specialists

A DIAGNOSIS of lupus means you have a chronic, life-long disease. It doesn't necessarily mean that you will die of it, but it does mean you need to assemble and maintain a good list of specialists for the syndromes and illnesses you will develop over time. It may be that your lupus is mild and the only specialist you'll ever need to use is your rheumatologist (see Day Two: Learning). It may be that your lupus is what is termed "severe," and you will end up needing a series of physicians, all specializing in different areas of the body that can be affected by lupus.

Let's take a look at what those doctors can do for you, how to assemble a team that can work together to keep you well, and what areas of the body may be affected by lupus during your lifetime.

While you read this chapter, keep in mind that everyone's lupus manifests in a different way: not all specialists will be needed by everyone, and not all areas of the body that *can* be affected by lupus will necessarily be affected in your case.

Is there a doctor in the house?

Specialists are medical doctors who have specialized in a particular field of medicine. They can be anything from foot doctors (podiatrists) to nose doctors (rhinologists). In your case, you have probably already gone to see a rheumatologist, which is a doctor specializing in rheumatological diseases, which includes SLE and other forms of lupus. Just like any medical doctor, specialists can be **board certified**, which means they have to pass medical board examinations as well as keep up to date on certain aspects of their field to continue their qualifications.

When looking for any specialist, ask if they are board certified in their specialty; this signifies a certain level of expertise that you will want from your physician. Some are certified as both internal medical doctors (**internists**—not to be confused with medical students who intern) and in their specialty. A high recommendation is that your PCP (primary care physician) be an internist, not just a regular M.D. Why? Internists are board certified and often have specialized in a specific field during their residency, which may relate to your lupus. In my case, my PCP is an internal medicine doctor who did a special rotation in rheumatology. I couldn't ask for a better fit!

As you and your rheumatologist discover the various ways in which your body responds to lupus, you will begin to draw a picture of what collection of specialists you will need at your disposal. For a lupus patient, this often means having a:

- O pulmonologist (lungs & blood circulation)
- O cardiologist (heart)
- O endocrinologist (endocrine & lymphatic system)
- O dermatologist (skin)
- O orthopedist (bones & connective muscles)
- O ophthalmologist (eyes)
- O neurologist (central nervous system)

This list is not meant to be exhaustive, but is simply a beginning point for you to consider. You and your PCP and/or rheumatologist will know when you need a specialist, and recommendations (and necessary insurance referrals) will be made at that time.

Finding a specialist entails not just blindly accepting a doctor that is recommended by your PCP, but finding out if that doctor can:

○ work well with other specialists
○ coordinate with your PCP
○ be open with you about your diagnoses and treatment
○ be someone you trust and feel comfortable working with
○ listen to your symptoms and offer adequate care as needed

I can't emphasize enough that you are in charge in the doctor–patient relationship, no matter the circumstances. This means *you* have to feel confident in and comfortable with your specialist. We have been trained, especially in America—and even more especially if we are women—that the doctor–patient relationship is akin to the adult–child relationship, with the doctor in the adult role. That leaves us with the role of being the child: uneducated, naïve, and helpless.

That isn't the way it works in reality, no matter what they're teaching in medical school. It's your illness; it's your doctor; you're in the driver's seat. If you are not confident you're receiving adequate care, or if you feel that your specialist is ignoring your reports of symptoms to the detriment of your health—get another specialist. *You're in charge.*

On the other side of the issue, be aware you may have read a lot about your disease, but your doctor is a board-certified specialist for a reason: she or he really is an expert in the field. You can learn a great deal from a specialist, given the right circumstances and the right doctor. Give the specialist a chance before deciding to find another one. Talk to them about any questions you may have. You may have a physician who opens up once you start asking questions rather than waiting for them to feed you information like a baby bird. Communication goes both ways in any relationship, including the doctor–patient one.

Finding a specialist that is right for you is rather like finding a mate: a good fit is hard to find, but once you find it, it can be one of the best things that ever happened to you.

Playing well with others

One of the biggest challenges when a team of specialists deals with one lupus patient is getting them to coordinate. Specialists are doctors with more years of training than usual under their belts; this can sometimes mean an even bigger than usual doctor's ego. And when egos are involved, cooperation among peers sometimes falls by the wayside.

One of the bulleted suggestions above about finding a specialist notes that the specialist in question should be able to work with other specialists. Another point was that the specialist should be able to coordinate with your primary care physician. These are very important issues when choosing a doctor for any one specialty. If your rheumatologist can't get information about your latest bout of pleurisy from your pulmonologist, and your PCP can't get all of *that* information, plus more, from your rheumatologist, chaos can ensue.

The necessary steps toward coordinating all the specialists often fall on the patient nowadays, although historically it is your PCP's position to collect all the information from your ongoing special doctors. Finding a PCP who will gladly coordinate your specialists is a godsend—finding one is often difficult, but necessary for a lupus patient. It may mean finding a new PCP: this can be a tough decision to make, especially if you've been seeing the same doctor all your life. It's up to you, but your PCP will be armed with more medical knowledge on how to coordinate the various specialty information coming in from your doctors than you. He or she will be able to catch critical decisions that have been made by specialists that may or may not have been made in coordination with other specialists. When this includes medication that may interact with other medication you're taking, this could mean literally saving your life from a simple mistake.

Egos may be bruised in the process of shuffling around specialists and perhaps moving to different doctors. It's going to be a difficult process for all involved, but necessary and well worth it for you to receive the high quality of medical care you deserve. Don't be afraid to tell a doctor that things aren't working out for you and that you want to move to a different specialist. Let them know why you're moving (what isn't working for you); it may help them in future interactions with other lupus patients.

Patient advocacy

It may be that you'll end up needing help in communication with your specialist that your PCP isn't able to handle for one reason or another. Or perhaps you're worried that all the information a specialist may give you will confuse you and you'll forget to write it all down, or forget to ask the right questions while you're in his or her office. In some cases, you may have a problem with your specialist, but you want to try avenues to solve your problems before moving to another doctor. In all these cases, the intermediary person brought in as a third party is referred to as a **patient advocate**.

Patient advocates can be professionals, such as nurses or staff at a hospital or doctor's office, or can be nonprofessionals, such as members of your family or friends. In the first instance, the professional advocate can be a person who works for you to help solve communication issues with your physicians. The professional patient advocate can also take on the role of being a conduit for questions and concerns you have for your specialist. A nonprofessional patient advocate is usually a family member or friend who accompanies you to the physician's office visits and helps you remember to ask the questions you had raised between visits, helps you remember symptoms that may have arisen lately, and helps you write down or remember information the specialist gives to you during visits.

Because lupus often carries chronic fatigue and what we lupus patients fondly refer to as "lupus fog," having a family member or friend help you sort out all the questions and information from all the various specialists can be a great help. Keep a notebook handy for all this information, too; both you and your patient advocate need to know where it's located and keep it up to date.

Because laws vary in different states regarding patient confidentiality, a nonfamily member may have a slightly more complicated time being your patient advocate. You may need to have a release signed to allow them access to your doctor's visits, and/or you may need to add them to a list (sometimes a legal document) which assigns them **medical power of attorney** in case of your inability to make medical decisions for yourself due to accident or incapacitating illness.

Durable medical power of attorney & advance directives

Having a medical power of attorney and what are called "**advance directives**" is a good idea for anyone. Advance directives give specific information to the hospital staff on how you would like to be treated in case of severe injury or illness that leaves you in a chronic vegetative or nonresponsive state. Ask at your local hospital for an advance directives form, and make sure a copy is on file at all local hospitals and all your doctors' offices. In an emergency, these offices and hospitals won't necessarily have time to contact each other to track down your paperwork; be sure everyone has copies, and you'll have a better chance that your wishes will be followed, even if you're incapacitated.

The same goes for your medical power of attorney documents. These give your person or people of choice the ability to make medical decisions in your name while you are incapacitated by illness or injury. Make sure all your local hospitals and your various doctors' offices have copies of it, and your patient advocate will be able to act on your behalf if you're not able to respond on your own behalf.

You can get more information about advance directives at the American Medical Association (AMA) Web site: http://www.ama-assn.org/public/booklets/livgwill.htm

More information on durable medical power of attorney can be found through your local legal aid or at the National Institutes of Health

(NIH) Web site: http://www.nlm.nih.gov/medlineplus/ency/article/001908.htm

Be aware that durable medical power of attorney forms differ from state to state. Check with an attorney in your state before filling out any "generic" forms.

IN A SENTENCE:

> *You need to assemble a good team of specialists and doctors who can work both with you and together to keep you healthy.*

learning

SLE-Related Syndromes and Conditions

LUPUS IS often not a solitary creature. It seems to like cohabiting with other related syndromes and conditions, all affecting different areas of the body, usually to do with the connective tissues, since lupus is a connective tissue disease. Lupus itself affects so many areas of the body that a team of specialists is usually necessary in order to treat all the conditions that may occur over the lifetime of a lupus patient.

Major areas of the body affected

Although lupus is a rheumatoid disease, unlike rheumatoid arthritis it tends to affect the connective tissues rather than the bones and joints. Connective tissue includes skin, muscles, tendons, internal organs, and **myofascia**. Think of myofascia as the connective tissue between skin, muscles, organs, and even your spinal column—it occurs, like packing material, between other tissues of your body. Later, in Day Six, we'll look into **Myofascial Pain Syndrome**

(**MPS**) and how it can combine with fibromyalgia as related syndromes that often affect lupus patients but can also occur on their own.

Along with myofascia, all the areas of connective tissue in the body are affected, including the major systems of the body: muscular, cardio-vascular, digestive, genitourinary, respiratory, central nervous system, and integumentary (connective tissues, including blood).

The sidebar on the facing page shows a simple chart of some areas of the body affected by lupus, along with some syndromes that can bring on these conditions.

When to turn to specialists

One of the most difficult learning curves in lupus is recognizing when you need to turn to medical doctors and/or when you need to see a specialist. Learning to recognize a flare or upcoming flare is difficult, as we've already discussed. On top of that, you will need to recognize when you need to turn to doctors in specialized areas of medicine for your needs.

Depending on your medical insurance situation, you may need to have recommendations or referrals made for you to see a specialist. If possible, talk to your primary care physician and set up referrals to the specialists you know you need to see on an ongoing basis, such as your rheumatologist or pulmonologist. Keep those referrals up to date, so you can call and make appointments as necessary when a flare of, say, pleurisy or severe tendonitis hits. Because lupus conditions often flare up without much warning, you will sometimes need to see a specialist in a hurry—keeping up your referrals and maintaining contact with your needed specialists is important in these situations.

Determining when you need to see a specialist as versus your primary care physician is something you need to discuss and sort out with your PCP on an ongoing basis. Some physicians feel proprietary about their patients and don't like them to see specialists unless it's absolutely nec-essary. On the other hand, some physicians would rather their lupus patients be aware of specialized needs, such as pulmonary, and go to the

Major Areas of the Body Affected by Lupus

Part of Body Affected	Complaint
Skin	○ lesions
	○ exema
	○ lupus (malar) "rash"
	○ discoid rash
	○ sunlight sensitivity
	○ mouth/nose ulcers
Organs	○ pleurisy (lungs)
	○ pericarditis & endocarditis (heart)
	○ kidney disease
	○ IBS (Irritable Bowel Syndrome) & other digestive syndromes
Blood	○ DVT (deep vein thrombosis, or blood clot)
	○ Lupus Anticoagulant Factor
Central Nervous System	○ seizures
	○ tremors
	○ migraines
	○ "brain fog"
	○ CNS lupus (affects brain & nervous system generally)
	○ sciatica
Muscles	○ tendonitis
	○ generalized muscular pain (akin to fibromyalgia pain, or accompanied by FM)

pulmonologist rather than seeing the regular physician first, only to need a referral to the pulmonologist for care—these physicians feel it's a waste of your time and theirs to go back and forth before you finally get treated.

Because the relationship with your various physicians is a very personal one, you need to tread carefully and keep the lines of communication open. Just as it's important to find specialists and primary care physicians who can collaborate well with each other, it's important for you to do the same and coordinate with your PCP to make sure his or her toes aren't getting stepped on if you go straight to a specialist for a certain condition, rather than going to your PCP for treatment.

Many lupus conditions don't necessarily demand specialist treatment, especially if your PCP is trained in handling lupus patients. Talk it through with your doctor as peers; he or she should be able to give you an idea as to when you want to seek specialized treatment as versus coming into the regular doctor's office when you have a flare-up of your illness.

When to call your doctor

Finally, you need to know when to call for medical attention in general. As lupus patients, we tend to become very self-informed about our condition. We read a lot of books (such as this one), materials from the various lupus foundations and support groups, and information from the Internet. All the information in the world can't compare to trained medical care, however.

When certain conditions flare up from lupus, such as tendonitis, generalized muscle pain, or even edema (fluid retention, such as in the legs or feet), we tend to take care of ourselves by following general guidelines for care. We elevate our feet, we take Tylenol for pain, we soak in a nice hot bath. But we can't always rely on our own treatments for lupus conditions. We need to recognize when it's time to call the doctor.

You can't rely on lists of symptoms to let you know when to call for an appointment or even for when to go to the emergency room. If in doubt, call your local hospital "ask a nurse" or your doctor immediately if you feel your symptoms are life-threatening. There are, however, certain signs you should never ignore:

○ Difficulty breathing
○ Sudden chest pain or pain down your arm accompanied by "heartburn"
○ Sudden swelling of a foot or ankle (or both) and pain in your leg (often behind the knee)
○ Sudden change in vision
○ Headache that won't go away
○ Seizure or sudden tremors
○ Inability to rouse from sleep (obviously someone else is going to have to call, in this case)
○ Bleeding that won't stop
○ Numbness or tingling that occurs suddenly and doesn't go away

There are many more such symptoms, too numerous to list here. For more information, talk to your primary care physician about your particular conditions.

For most lupus patients, the same syndromes and illnesses will occur over and over again (such as an annual bout of pleurisy or tendonitis), making it easier for both patients and physicians to predict what conditions will need treatment by medical doctors and what conditions can be treated at home by the patients when flares occur.

IN A SENTENCE:

> *Learning to know when to call your doctor or a specialist is key to maintaining good health for the lupus patient.*

living

Fibromyalgia and Systemic Lupus

FIBROMYALGIA IS distinct from lupus but is often either mistaken for it before a definitive diagnosis is made, or is carried along with it by people who have lupus. Fibromyalgia (sometimes referred to simply as FM) confers a great deal of pain on its sufferers, and although it is not as medically threatening to the entire body as lupus, its chronic pain is nothing to be ignored or downplayed. Proper diagnosis of fibromyalgia and treatment of its symptoms are key to living with this syndrome, whether the patient has it alone or carries it along with systemic lupus.

Living with pain

Fibromyalgia is a noninflammatory, nonprogressive, chronic syndrome characterized by pain in muscles and tendons and the myofascial tissues connecting muscle groups, marked by a series of tender spots throughout the body in a synchronous pattern (see diagram under the Learning section of this chapter). A flare-up of fibromyalgia can result in a patient feeling as if she wants to simply lie still in bed and sleep. Other symptoms include fatigue, sleep disturbance, depression (from pain and lack of sleep, primarily), broken and curved fingernails, flulike achiness, and temperature fluctuations in the body.

The pain caused by fibromyalgia can range from a generalized achiness to high levels of pain that can incapacitate the patient. A life lived in pain is a difficult one, both for the patient and for those who comprise his or her support group. Living with that pain is the goal of a fibromyalgia sufferer—but living with pain is certainly doable.

Pain control can take any number of avenues. Many books have been written about living with pain, as well as many specifically about fibromyalgia. My intention here is to give you some high points on pain control and living with fibromyalgia; even if you don't have this particular syndrome, pain control and various coping techniques for muscle pain can be applied to muscle and myofascial pain found otherwise in lupus. This isn't meant to be a complete course on either pain or FM, but rather an overview from the standpoint of someone, myself, who has fibromyalgia as well as a number of lupus-related conditions, and within the venue of how it can affect a lupus patient.

Pain and cortisol

Pain and stress responses both stimulate the production of cortisol. One of the findings from recent research into fibromyalgia is that patients with the syndrome don't produce cortisol in normal quantities. Pain may be a way of the body responding to this lack. Research into the way the adrenal gland produces cortisol, and the way cortisol then interacts with the body to stop pain—in sufficient quantities—or create pain—when in insufficient quantities—is being done at various hospitals under the aegis of studies by the National Institutes of Health (National Institute of Arthritis and Musculoskeletal and Skin Diseases). More information on those studies can be found online at http://www.nih.gov/niams/healthinfo/fibrofs.htm.

Cortisol is also created when a person is under stress; for the same reasons we want lupus patients to stay on a low-stress course, we want fibromyalgia patients to do the same in order to lower their pain levels.

A lovely woman I know, who owns her own business locally, has restructured her life in order to reduce stress because of her fibromyalgia. By focusing her business on the basic core of her services, pulling back from expansions she had made in the last few years, she has been able to reduce the role pain plays in her life. Because of the lessened pain, she's not only able to live a more full life with fibromyalgia, but she's been able to increase her business within her focused area without stressing herself.

Lowering pain levels

Ask your doctor about seeing a pain specialist: often these are found at your local hospital in a pain clinic, and are usually anesthesiologists trained specifically in pain control and techniques to help you cope (not just mechanical methods, either!). These specialists can help you learn to live with fibromyalgia and chronic pain by teaching pain control methods.

Pain control can be done by two methods: *mental* and *mechanical.*

LOWERING PAIN MENTALLY

Mental methods of pain control include:

○ meditation
○ self-hypnosis
○ biofeedback
○ visualization techniques
○ positive support

Most areas of the U.S., Canada, and Western Europe have support groups available for fibromyalgia (sometimes referred to by its older name, fibrosytis), often at local hospitals, rehabilitation clinics, and health organizations such as the visiting nurses association. These groups teach and support FM patients on various mental techniques to cope with chronic pain. Take advantage of learning formally how to meditate and produce positive feedback to control pain; visualization techniques can help you control your pain both when it occurs and in order to stave off daily stress that might otherwise cause a flare-up of fibromyalgia pain.

The positive support of a group of other fibromyalgia patients will also help you reduce stress, lower your pain levels, and learn to cope mentally with the pain you do endure as an FM patient.

LOWERING PAIN MECHANICALLY

Mechanical methods of coping with pain from fibromyalgia include:

- swimming-pool therapy
- nonweight-bearing exercise
- massage
- acupuncture & acupressure
- medications
- rest

Ask your primary care physician or rheumatologist about a referral for supervised swimming-pool therapy and/or nonweight-bearing exercise with a local clinic or rehabilitation center. Ideally, one should be located that has at least one physical therapist who has specialized training in working with FM patients. There has been some debate in the past about rest versus exercise for reducing pain in fibromyalgia patients, but it has been found that gentle exercise in nonweight-bearing surroundings, such as a swimming pool, has had beneficial results for not only reducing stress and existing pain, but training the muscles to resist future pain by stimulating their proper use in a controlled environment.

Massage can include a newer form called myofascial massage. This works the myofascial areas connecting the muscles, rather than the muscles themselves. Recently, it has been shown to provide relief from pain without stimulating the muscles to tighten or produce more pain. Ask your physician or physical therapist about the possibility of receiving such massage, rather than the "regular" sort of massage one can get from any qualified/licensed massage therapist.

Acupuncture and its lighter cousin, acupressure, are gaining in popularity as well as acceptance in standard medical circles for both coping with and reducing pain. Check with your medical insurance company to see if you may qualify for these therapies if you are interested in exploring nontraditional, non-Western methods for dealing with pain. I have personally been seeing an acupuncturist for pain relief for the last year and can attest to its efficacy on a subjective level—I can tell when I've missed some appointments with Jeanne Ann, as my pain levels rise again.

On a more traditional note, pain medications are also of use with fibromyalgia; don't let anyone fool you into thinking that you're a "sissy" for not being able to handle large levels of pain from fibromyalgia without aid, either mental or mechanical. As far as medications go, check with your physician and talk about options—there are many modern formulations that can help with the specific pain found in FM without making you become dependent on drugs or dopey from side effects. If you are seeing a pain specialist, he or she should be of great help in advising you about medications available for your specific needs, both short- and long-term.

Finally, rest and relaxation are a mechanical response that is needed in balance to the exercise mentioned previously. Just as you must recognize an upcoming flare of lupus, you need to recognize what will cause an FM flare and head it off at the pass by resting when necessary. This doesn't mean becoming a couch potato—believe me, it's an easy mistake to fall into. "Oh, I'm in pain, so I can't move," becomes the mantra, and sooner than you think, you can end up gaining weight, becoming more immobile through the disuse of muscles and joints, and putting yourself in a cycle of pain and immobility that is hard to break. On the other hand, you need to pace your exercise carefully so as not to end up *needing* rest in order to recover from your exertions. Just as living with lupus requires a delicate balance, living with fibromyalgia requires that same knife-edge of life walked between pain and wellness.

Coping methods

Coping with pain is just as important as controlling it and can be done via the methods listed above, plus a boost of support from your local (or online) support group. Coping also means living with pain without making those around you miserable.

It's hard to live with pain and not make those around you aware that it exists, but the stress of seeing you in pain causes (mental) pain to those who love you. They *know* you're in pain because they know you have a chronic syndrome that is characterized by pain. What they don't necessarily need to know is every ache and twinge you experience. And learning how to mask those twinges is something you may want to learn how to do. Just as professional athletes learn the difference between "good pain" and "bad pain," you too must learn how to differentiate between normal (for fibromyalgia) pain, and pain that signifies something more serious or a new condition.

How do you do this? By learning to listen to yourself and also learning how your responses to pain are characterized by your physical posture, facial expressions, and speech patterns. Videotaping yourself while you're in pain may help: watch how you hold yourself when you're in pain. Do you lean forward? Rock on your heels? Unconsciously clutch at the limb that's hurting? Do you squinch your face up, or twitch your mouth *just so*, or blink more often? They may be small signals, but signals nonetheless, and those who are close to you will learn to recognize them even before you do. You may want to ask your spouse, significant other, or even a close friend for help in identifying these signals: explain that you don't want to *hide* your pain, but you want to learn how to cope with it by learning its signals.

Sometimes we signal our pain to others without even realizing we're in pain at the time: learning these signals means learning to recognize our own pain and how we're suppressing its signals to our brains.

While writing this book, my good friend, Bruce Hadley has been working on building an addition between my house and barn. While helping him out, he's had to say to me on more than one occasion, "Nancy, you need to take a break now." I was making small but recognizable "Nancy in Pain" facial expressions and body postures without even realizing it. Bad me. I need to listen to my own advice!

Don't ignore your pain—pain that is outside your "normal" parameters of FM pain can mean something serious is happening. Learn to listen to your body and the variations between your different types of pain. This isn't an easy thing to do, as I can attest to myself, but the goal is to reduce stress not only for yourself but your support group.

IN A SENTENCE:

> *You can learn to control and reduce pain levels through mental and mechanical methods, supported by friends' and family's input.*

learning

What Is Fibromyalgia?

ACCORDING TO the National Institutes of Health (NIH), fibromyalgia is "a chronic disorder characterized by widespread musculoskeletal pain, fatigue, and multiple tender points." It is classified with rheumatological diseases and syndromes, much as lupus is, but unlike lupus it is not inflammatory or degenerative. It ebbs and wanes in "flares" like its sister rheumatological syndromes, and may or may not be triggered by an accident or illness that sets it off in the first place. For myself, fibromyalgia started after I broke my back in a riding accident in 1988 (just compression fractures, thank goodness); the jury remains out on whether or not that was a coincidence or a cause.

What causes fibromyalgia?

No one knows what causes fibromyalgia, though it may be linked to a predisposition genetically, like lupus, then triggered by an incident, as noted above. Or it may be triggered by a virus, since certain post-Lyme disease syndromes resemble fibromyalgia to a great degree (research in this area is ongoing currently through the NIH).

Since its first description in 1816 by William Balfour, a Scottish physician, fibromyalgia (or fibrosytis) was thought to be a mental disorder wherein the patient created pain for him or herself. In 1987, the American Medical Association (AMA) finally recognized it as a separate and valid syndrome. Some physicians, unfortunately, still view it as primarily a mental process rather than a physical condition. It goes without saying that you will want to find a physician who is *not* of that opinion, if you want to receive adequate treatment for your fibromyalgia.

What are trigger points?

Fibromyalgia presents with tender points in bilateral areas of the body, both above and below the waist, and on the limbs. In order to qualify as a fibromyalgia patient, you need to show tenderness in a certain number of these points, at least 11 out of the 18 shown on the diagram on the opposite page, and general pain throughout the body for at least three months prior to diagnosis. The trigger points need to be tender on both sides of the body, in a symmetrical pattern, and in all four quadrants (upper and lower, right and left).

Now, I'm sure you're muttering to yourself, "If someone pokes me hard enough, I'd be tender *anywhere*." True enough, but when the rheumatologist or PCP tests you for trigger point tenderness, they will use gentle pressure—although, if you have fibromyalgia, this pressure will feel a great deal stronger than it really is. When I say *tender,* I mean TENDER. Fibromyalgia patients will often jump when a point is touched even lightly, if they're in flare.

What causes tenderness at the trigger points? It seems to be a combination of myofascial pain (not to be confused with Myofascial Pain Syndrome, though it's related) and points where the joints and ligaments connect. All doctors know about fibromyalgia is that it causes pain throughout the body, and sometimes carries the following conditions along with it:

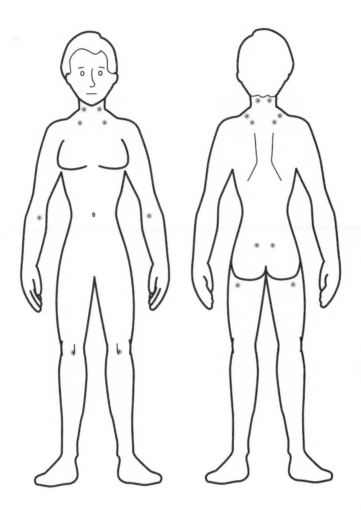

- ○ fatigue
- ○ IBS (irritable bowel syndrome)
- ○ sleep disorder
- ○ headaches
- ○ cognitive impairment (including memory problems, like "brain fog")
- ○ chemical sensitivities
- ○ sensitivity to bright light, sound, and smells

A very general statement could be this in short: Having fibromyalgia is being *sensitive* all over your body.

Myofascial Pain Syndrome

MPS is a syndrome that is usually seen hand-in-hand with fibromyalgia and is, sometimes, simply categorized along with it instead of as a separate condition.

In the case of myofascial pain, the connective tissues between muscles, organs, and bones becomes painful and causes ropey, knotted muscles that are obvious on the patient's body. Where fibromyalgia shows no inflamed muscles, MPS will show knots on your body that can be responsive to regular massage, as well as myofascial massage techniques.

No one knows what causes myofascial pain, just as no one knows what causes fibromyalgia, unfortunately. Treatment for MPS is about the same as it is for FM, which is why so many doctors categorize them together. While fibromyalgia seems to be caused by neurotransmitters misfiring pain indicators, MPS is a skeletal-muscular disorder —many times, it is triggered by injury, overworked muscle groups, sleep disturbances (causing muscles to fail to relax properly during sleep), or repetitive motions.

How can fibromyalgia be treated?

Treatments, as we've discussed in the Living section of this day, consist of a combination of both mental and mechanical means of controlling and preventing pain. The other key is a balance of rest and relaxation alongside gentle, nonweight-bearing exercise (such as in a swimming pool). It all comes down to *balance*—that seems to be the key not only with lupus but also with fibromyalgia. All of these chronic, pain-giving diseases require us to be vigilant about being aware of our bodies and the symptoms we experience, and to learn to balance our lives with rest and exercise, in measure, so we can stave off flares of pain or illness.

No wonder it's so much work to live with lupus and its sister syndromes!

IN A SENTENCE:

> *Fibromyalgia is a syndrome of musculoskeletal pain in a pattern of trigger points throughout the body.*

DAY **7**

living

Chronic Fatigue

ONE OF the biggest "gotchas" of lupus is the fatigue factor. When a flare hits, it is sometimes heralded by a wave of fatigue, tiredness, and soreness, often as if you're coming down with the flu. By this time, you've learned about lupus in general and some of the areas of the body affected by lupus, as well as at least one of the syndromes that's often carried along with or mistaken for lupus. Now, at the end of the first week—post-diagnosis—we're going to start looking at some of the effects of lupus on your life, in this case, the role fatigue is going to play in your life from now on.

I'm always exhausted

Clinical fatigue, as versus regular tiredness, is a bone-deep exhaustion that doesn't abate for weeks at a time. You will feel exhausted as soon as you try to move around, perhaps even while you're sitting still. You will fall asleep in the middle of sentences, or lose what you were about to say because your mind drifted off. You will often wake in the morning (if you can get up before the afternoon!) feeling as if you didn't get a good night's sleep and still be tired. Coffee and tea won't make you feel any more awake—though they may give you the jitters.

You're going to feel as if you're not getting enough done; you'll need naps often. Worst of all, even your most supportive family members and friends may not understand your fatigue sufficiently and act as if you're just "being lazy." Explaining clinical fatigue to them will sometimes be a difficult prospect, but you need to help them understand. *You're not being lazy.* What you're experiencing is a medical reality, and although it isn't always obvious to the naked eye, it's because you have a very real disease and this exhaustion is a very real component of that disease.

Have your support network of friends and family read up on Chronic Fatigue Syndrome (CFS). Although what you are experiencing is *not* CFS, the symptoms are very similar because both fatigues are classified as **clinical chronic fatigue**. In other words, both lupus fatigue and CFS are fatigues that are persistent (chronic) and can be diagnosed clinically by a medical doctor. Treatment for lupus fatigue differs from that of CFS to a great degree, because your exhaustion is stemming from your body attacking its own self. In CFS's case, no one really knows what causes it, but it appears to be from a virus or group of viruses that attack the immune system and actually cause immunodeficiency. What you have, instead, is an overly active immune system. Strange, isn't it, how both ends of the same spectrum of immune conditions create clinical fatigue? It's the body's response to its delicate balance being out of whack.

Unfortunately, most texts and articles about lupus don't go into any detail about clinical fatigue, leading to more misunderstandings both by patients and friends and family—everyone ends up wondering what's going on. But unlike the fatigue associated with lupus, information on CFS is easily found both in books and on the Internet, and can reassure your support group that you are not being lazy: you have clinical fatigue and it can and will be treated. But most of all, they need to understand that you're going to have both good and bad days.

Bad days

Lupus is a disease that ebbs and flows. You'll have good, healthy times, and you'll have flare-ups that will leave you sick and perhaps even in the hospital. These same flares are often presaged by fatigue moving in. That's when the "bad days" can start up.

Little can be done about these bad days except to ride them out. I know from my own experience that a balance of rest and exercise has to be maintained even through the fatigue, hard though that may be. The trick is knowing when enough is enough, and catching yourself before it becomes too much. Too much may, on a bad day, be walking out to the mailbox down that quarter-mile driveway you have in the country. On a good day, you could do it easily, though it might wear you down a bit. But on a bad day, if you drag yourself, fatigued and exhausted, up and down that driveway, you might end up causing the lupus flare to be exaggerated. Instead, try asking someone else to get the mail, but make yourself sit down and sort it at the dining room table. That may be enough before you need to make lunch, then have a nap.

Only you know what is "enough," and only time will give you enough experience to be able to predict what that is. For some people, a bad day of lupus fatigue means they can only golf nine holes. For others, sorting the mail puts them in bed for a few hours. Listen to your body, but remember that you need to be practical about your fatigue. You can't live in bed forever. You may be able to do more than you think if you keep a positive outlook.

POSITIVE REINFORCEMENT

I know this sounds Pollyanna-ish, but it's true. Positive visualizations, repetition of positive motivations, have been proven by medical science to improve all sorts of conditions, including cancer. In the case of chronic fatigue, take a few minutes on a morning of a "bad day" and say to yourself, "I'm going to have a good day today. I'm going to feel energized and happy. I look good, I feel good, and I'm going to accomplish

————- (fill in one accomplishment you want to make today)." Then strive for that goal without thinking that you have to drag yourself through the day to get it done. It can be a small goal. Then, when that's done, promise yourself a slightly bigger one the next day.

One source of help may be reading the FlyLady's Web site (www.flylady.com). This is a woman who has revolutionized cleaning the house into small steps that can be done in 15 minutes a day. She's a great inspiration, and her techniques can be used for anything—not just housecleaning. I've used it for my business, for writing, for all sorts of things. Her Web site allows you to sign up—free—for e-mail reminders and newsletters, all constructed to help you use her methods to break down what seem to be overwhelming tasks into small steps you can do in a short amount of time with little energy.

I've had a great deal of clinical fatigue while writing this book because, goodness knows, writing can be a stressful if unathletic process. What I've done is set myself a goal of a certain number of words a day to write, knowing how many words I can write in so many hours. When I feel I've accomplished that goal and don't feel exhausted from it, I up the ante and set myself a slightly higher goal. By doing this, I've been able to push myself through more writing with less stress simply by *telling myself I can do it*. It's amazing what the mind can do to help the body overcome fatigue.

This is not to say that a bad day is not going to put you on your back in bed. It will, eventually. It happens to me more often than I'm willing to admit. There will be days all the positive thoughts in the world can't overcome. And that's *normal*. Don't beat yourself up with the thought that you've failed somehow if you can't beat the fatigue all the time. You can't. You're human, and sometimes the lupus wins out. In those cases, rest is what's called for.

Home and work compromises

Compromises are going to have to be made—there's no way around it. You have lupus, and living with this disease means a life of compromise, to a greater or lesser extent. We can always hope it will be lesser!

As I discussed in Day Four, adjusting your lifestyle to reduce stress is a key to controlling your flare-ups of lupus. In the same way, adjusting your home and work lifestyles will be key to controlling your fatigue, since it often comes with or just before a flare occurs.

Go back to Day Four and take a look at the chart on page 39. Look at what activities you do at what times of the day and how your response to them corresponds to stress levels. Now do the same chart again, but this time I want you to note how your *energy feels* during different times of the day with different levels of activity (next page). For the best results you should do this chart several times, particularly on good days and bad days: days you feel you have good energy levels and days you feel you are fatigued.

Now I want you to determine what activities at what time of the day are making you tired on a consistent basis. It may be that your fatigue is triggered by activities in the evening or morning; or you may get tired in the afternoon without any activity at all. If it helps, plot a chart of your up- and down-swings of energy, like the chart below.

What we're trying to determine is whether it is particular activities, times of the day, or a combination of the two that are aggravating your clinical fatigue. When you have a good idea as to what worsens your

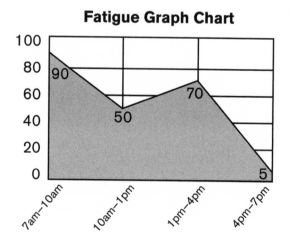

Fatigue Graph Chart

Fatigue Diary

TIME	ACTIVITY: What, where, with whom	ENERGY LEVELS 1–5: 1=energized, 2=normal, 3=tired, 4=very tired, 5=exhausted
7am		
8am		
9am		
10am		
11am		
Noon		
1pm		
2pm		
3pm		
4pm		
5pm		
6pm		
7pm		
8pm		
9pm		
10pm		
11pm		

fatigue, then you can go about making a list of ways you may stave off these fatigue peaks. Just as you modified your lifestyle in Day Four to accommodate stress levels, you will need to do the same to accommodate your fatigue. Stress, in fact, causes fatigue, too.

Talk to your family and your friends and see if you can get them to help with certain activities to lessen your fatigue. If you find you are now a "night person" rather than a morning person, see if you can be the one to fix dinner, but have your spouse or roommate do breakfast. Many lupus patients find, in fact, that their energy rises at night, rather than in the morning, making them into night owls. Job accommodations may need to be made for just this situation, as well. Can you switch to a night shift? Can you float your hours to come in late and leave late?

You may want to choose the high-energy point of the day (or night) to do your most mentally challenging activities, as fatigue causes brain fog in a big way. It's difficult to think clearly when you're constantly falling asleep. Even if you seem to feel okay, you may actually not be thinking as clearly as you'd like to during certain parts of the day; keep that in mind when you're making your chart and graph, above.

IN A SENTENCE:

> By learning what triggers your chronic fatigue, you can modify your lifestyle and use positive reinforcement to live a more active life.

learning

Clinical Fatigue

CLINICAL CHRONIC fatigue differs from simple fatigue by its very definition: it is fatigue that is clinically defined by a medical professional and lasts for longer than a few weeks, making it chronic. It's important to define clinical fatigue as well as how it is diagnosed and treated, to assure you, the lupus patient, that what you're experiencing is a real medical condition and not just "sleepiness" or "laziness."

What is clinical chronic fatigue?

Clinical fatigue is an overwhelming tiredness and fatigue that does not respond to standard medications for other conditions that create fatigue—such as depression—which lasts for more than three weeks at a time. Clinical chronic fatigue is that same tiredness that lasts for a long time and then comes back, or never leaves, making it into a chronic, persistent state.

Only a physician can diagnose clinical fatigue. He or she will test for various conditions that could cause such fatigue, to rule them out, such as:

- depression
- Chronic Fatigue Syndrome (often caused by the Epsom-Barr virus)
- adrenal gland imbalance
- thyroid gland imbalance
- narcolepsy
- sleep disturbances

    - insomnia
    - restless leg syndrome
    - sleep apnea
    - gastrointestinal reflux

If none of these conditions test positively, then your doctor will probably diagnose clinical chronic fatigue associated with lupus.

How can fatigue be treated?

Various treatments for lupus-induced chronic fatigue can be explored between you and your primary care physician or rheumatologist. Just as I discussed earlier in this chapter, you can handle fatigue only to a limited extent through mental means of positive reinforcement. Telling yourself that you can push through to a goal only goes so far. From that point on, you may need to talk about medications that can help your condition and let you lead a normal lifestyle both at home and in the workplace.

One medication that is often used in treating lupus is hydroxychloroquine, which is usually known by its brand name, **Plaquenil**. This is an **antimalarial** drug that has been used with great success in managing rheumatoid arthritis. We'll talk in more detail about this drug in Week Two. For now, we want to focus on Plaquenil's beneficial side effect, which is that it seems to help with fatigue to a great extent. Many patients who have lupus, and many who have Sjögren's Syndrome (see Months Two and Four), have reported relief from tiredness and chronic fatigue by taking Plaquenil daily. Side effects of Plaquenil unfortunately preclude a small number of people from taking it—I'm one of the few, in fact.

For those of us who can't take Plaquenil, there are some other options for medications. One is azathioprine, or Imuran. This is an **immunosuppressant** drug that is used rarely and carefully, as it suppresses the immune system response of the patient. Blood tests must be taken every six to eight weeks to monitor liver, kidney, and white blood cell levels, to make sure the immune system isn't being suppressed too much. On the other hand, Imuran often helps with chronic fatigue, allowing patients who have overwhelming fatigue to lead more normally active lives. Immunosuppressants have serious side effects and are usually only explored by your rheumatologist if you have severe lupus that affects your internal organs or kidneys, combined with severe chronic fatigue.

By working with your doctor, and exploring a combination of medication and positive reinforcement, you can indeed live with chronic fatigue and still maintain a lifestyle that, while taking compromises into account, can be satisfying and reasonably active.

IN A SENTENCE:

> *Your doctor can diagnose chronic fatigue caused by lupus and treat it effectively, allowing you to become more active.*

FIRST-WEEK MILESTONE

At the end of week one, you've covered a lot of territory, learned a great deal, and experienced a range of emotions from relief to anger to denial and disbelief, and finally to acceptance.

By now you will have learned:

○ MAJOR CLINICAL INFORMATION ABOUT WHAT LUPUS IS, ITS DIFFERENT FORMS, WHAT MAY CAUSE LUPUS, AND COMMON TREATMENTS FOR THE DISEASE.

○ WHY LUPUS IS SO HARD TO DIAGNOSE AND WHY IT MAY HAVE TAKEN SO LONG FOR YOU TO GET A DIAGNOSIS.

○ HOW TO FIND A GOOD RHEUMATOLOGIST AND RECOGNIZE WHEN A FLARE OF LUPUS ILLNESS COULD COME ON.

○ HOW TO LOWER STRESS AT WORK AND HOME BY TRACKING YOUR ACTIVITIES.

○ WHAT SPECIALISTS CAN DO FOR YOU AND WHAT SPECIALISTS YOU'LL NEED TO ASSEMBLE.

- ○ ABOUT CHRONIC PAIN FROM A SISTER SYNDROME, FIBROMYALGIA.

- ○ TECHNIQUES FOR LOWERING PAIN AND CONTROLLING IT.

- ○ ABOUT CLINICAL CHRONIC FATIGUE.

You're on your way to living a full life with your lupus.

living

Drug Treatments
for Systemic Lupus

MOST TREATMENTS for lupus involve medications: yes, better living through chemistry. Drugs will be your friend. You'll hear all the jokes, as you take any number of pills a day, but the truth is that you'll be better off for taking a regime of vitamins, supplements, and the all-important medications that will be prescribed by your physician, rheumatologist, and other specialists.

During Week Two, you will learn how to handle those medications, how to reorganize your life around them, aid your support group in helping you with all these meds, what medications are commonly prescribed for lupus, and what these medications do to help you with your disease.

Beyond denial and depression: the importance of taking your medications

I take over sixteen different medications and supplements a day. No, that's not sixteen pills: sixteen actual medications. It adds up to over thirty pills a day, depending on how I'm doing, healthwise. That's a lot to handle, and it's a lot to wrap your mind around. And I'm not alone: I know a number of lupoids who take even more medications than I do. The main reason for this isn't the lupus *itself,* but the overlapping syndromes and conditions that arise from having a screwy immune system. One woman, for instance, will take medications for a slow digestive system, another set for lupus headaches, yet more for arthritis, and even more to prevent future blood clots.

It isn't unusual to take a look at the pile of pills each day and want to rebel, to just not take them. It's a normal reaction, and it's part of the denial process of lupus. Remember how in Week One we discussed the grief-cycle reaction to the diagnosis of lupus? That cycle doesn't end abruptly, just as it doesn't end in physical grief situations when you've lost a loved one. The responses of denial, anger, depression, resignation, and acceptance do *change* in that they manifest differently every time you go through the cycle of grief, but you will cycle again and again as you go through your life. Each cycle will, hopefully, be more short-lived and less intense.

It's a hard thing to say, but you need to get beyond your denial and your depression about having lupus and *take your medications.* Not taking them isn't going to make the disease go away, and in fact will probably exacerbate your symptoms. I'm sure you're saying to yourself, "I'd never think of not taking my pills. I'm good about following directions." Believe me, you *will* get to the point in your life, at least once, where you're sick and tired of being sick and tired, and all you want to do is ignore your medications—as if by ignoring them, they (and the lupus) will go away.

I know I sound like a broken record, but the fact is that ignoring your medications won't make your lupus go away. Take your pills!

Organizing your medications

One way to help in all this mess of pill-taking is good organization. You may not have to take as many supplements and medications as I do, so different methods will work better for different people.

Overall, you need either a daily or weekly pill box, one with adequate room for all your pills, including vitamins and minerals. Anything that you take throughout the day will go in the box. Most pharmacies have a section where you can find pill boxes that are organized by day (morning, afternoon, evening) or by week (daily), or sometimes even by month. Most pill boxes I've found can't hold the big vitamins, so I end up using the weekly boxes and spreading out the daily pills throughout the little compartments. I've then relabelled the compartments with tape so as to show my morning, afternoon, evening, and bedtime meds.

If you can't find a pill box that's big enough, you may need to make one for yourself or improvise. If you don't go out often, and usually take your medications at home, you may want to get some little glass custard cups from a supermarket or cooking store, label them appropriately with tape, and put your medications in them. Then nest the cups and place them on your kitchen table, so they're handy to find.

Fill your pill boxes or cups in the evening, before you go to bed, or first thing in the morning (if you're one of those morning people). That way you'll be all set for the day. If you have several pill boxes, you can even do a couple of days at a time!

If you have children or pets, never put your medications out where they can be easily handled by others—place them in a locked cabinet or a high place where only you can reach. Same goes for any pill box you may use, when it's not tucked away safely (unknown to little hands) in your purse or backpack or briefcase.

Even with a nicely organized pill box, you may still feel overwhelmed at all the medications staring at you throughout the day. If you feel overwhelmed, try this trick: Talk to your doctor and pharmacist about which pills need to be taken with meals and which can be taken on an empty stomach. If you have some in the morning cycle that can be taken alone, you may want to divide those off from the other morning pills and take them pre-breakfast with a cup of coffee or tea. That way you won't feel as overwhelmed by pills when you have your breakfast. Same for lunch or dinner, or even bedtime meds. See how you can spread them out throughout the day so you don't feel as if you're taking too many at once; beware, however, of spreading them out too far. You may end up feeling as though you are taking a never-ending flow of medications from morning till night!

And *always* check with your doctor and pharmacist before moving your medications around. *Never* move a medication from its time slot without talking to a medical professional first.

Use your support group

Don't forget your support group when it comes to taking and organizing your medications. If you have a supportive spouse, sibling, or friend, you might want to ask them to help you organize your medications as we discussed above. Having someone else in on the process often makes it easier, and less easy to deny the fact that you have all those pills to take.

The same goes for taking the pills themselves. If your support people are in on the game, they'll know that you are going to have days when you don't want to take your medications. I know myself pretty well, and when my husband goes away for any period of time, I ask a good friend to come over and check in on me. Part of the check is to make sure I've actually taken my medications—it's not that I've necessarily refused to take them, but subconsciously I can rather easily "forget" to take all those pills. It sounds silly, but it works. Just having someone drop in and ask over a cup of coffee, "So, did you take your pills this morning?" gets me motivated to do the Adult Thing and take my meds.

Surviving medications

Several lupus medications have difficult side effects; some more than others. One of the more difficult drugs is **corticosteroids**, particularly Prednisone. "Surviving" Prednisone is something many lupus patients have to endure.

When I say *survive,* I don't mean that the medication will likely kill you; what I mean is that getting through the side effects of having to take it is something you won't enjoy, and you need to learn how to survive through it. It's a drug that can literally save your life, but it's also harsh on both your body and your mind.

As we'll discuss in the next section of this chapter, Prednisone and all corticosteroids work by (1) depressing the immune system response, thereby (2) reducing inflammation in the connective tissues. Unlike pure **anti-inflammatories**, Prednisone, and its sister steroids, such as Medrol, work at reducing inflammation, but because of the way they affect the body, they also increase fat deposits and cause swelling in other areas. Prednisone creates the infamous "moon face" you often see in lupus patients. Your face becomes rounded: your cheeks round out like a chipmunk's; your eyes get puffy; your face is flushed red. If you're on a high enough dose for long enough, your breasts and stomach will get larger—I made a joke when I was on Prednisone for a protracted period of time that I looked like one of those ancient stone figures of the fertility goddess. More dangerous side effects can occur from Prednisone, as we'll see in the Learning section of this chapter.

All in all, though, corticosteroids can, as I said earlier, save your life. If your doctor wants you on a course of them for some life-threatening conditions of lupus, by all means don't argue, but if you think you may be on them for too long or for reasons you can't understand, discuss this with your doctor. It may be that she or he can wean you off the Prednisone and some of those side effects, such as the moon face, will eventually subside.

Losing weight while taking Prednisone is difficult; I won't downplay it. I continue to struggle with that issue, myself. Sometimes normal weight-loss plans won't work to get rid of the chest/stomach enlargement: talk to your doctor and see if she has some suggestions for a combination of diet and exercise to help.

IN A SENTENCE:

> *Medications will be a vital part of your life with lupus: it's important to take them diligently.*

learning

Lupus Medications and Their Effects

THERE ARE several different classes of medications commonly prescribed for lupus, including nonsteroidal anti-inflammatories (NSAIDs), antimalarials, chemotherapy (immunosuppressants), corticosteroids, and antidepressants. Various nutritional supplements are also recommended by most physicians.

The role of NSAIDs

Nonsteroidal anti-inflammatories (NSAIDs) are a class of drug that cause a decrease in inflammation response in the connective tissues without the use of corticosteroids. In other words, NSAIDs reduce "puffiness." This puffiness can be inflammation in any of your tissues, but in this case we're concerned about your connective tissues, including your organs, skin, and muscles/tendons. What NSAIDs do is work against or help block the chemical reaction in your body that the immune system creates in response to what it thinks is something bad. That response usually takes the form of inflammation. Because a lupus patient's immune system is hyperactive (works overtime), it thinks that perfectly normal things are "bad," and reacts by forming an inflammation that isn't really necessary. These inflammations can be anything from swollen glands to tendonitis (swollen tendons) to pneumonia.

Common NSAID brands used for lupus as of 2003 are:

- Celebrex
- Vioxx
- Advil
- Aleve
- Naprosyn
- Voltaren
- Daypro

One of the side effects of NSAIDs can be stomach upset or even the formation of ulcers, as they're harsh on the stomach lining. Many of the modern brands have time-release formulations to guard against this side effect, as well as calming agents to help ease any stomach upset. You can read more about your particular brand's side effects and chemical components in the current *PDR* (*Physicians Desk Reference*), often found in libraries, a current consumer drug manual (check your library, bookstore, or even supermarket), and online at WebMD (http://www. webmd.com).

NSAIDs are the number one medicine used in lupus because of the inflammation caused by the disease. They're also used in treating arthritis, which is often carried along with lupus, since it's a condition classified with rheumatoid arthritis. Your doctor will presumably try NSAIDs first in treating the symptoms of your lupus, including such conditions as tendonitis, pleurisy, arthritis, and generalized swelling of tissues or muscles. Since NSAIDs have the least amount of side effects and the greatest efficacy in treating the most common forms and effects of lupus, they will probably be a mainstay in your medicine cabinet from now on.

Antimalarials

Another mainstay of lupus medicine is the group of antimalarial drugs commonly used to treat rheumatoid arthritis. The most popular antimalarial brand name is Plaquenil, which is a form of hydroxychloroquine. What this drug basically does is trick the body into thinking you have a low-level form of malaria, and the body turns its attention to that, instead of doing its usual lupus trick of attacking perfectly good tissue. Some of the common side effects from Plaquenil, therefore, are low fevers and diarrhea, especially until your body gets used to the medicine.

I made the mistake of starting up Plaquenil for the first time and then heading off to an outdoors, all-day Highland Games at Loon Mountain, NH. If only I had listened to my doctor's advice to "take it easy" for the first week! I spent the day rushing in and out of every Port-A-Potty on the games' site. At least I stayed dry when it rained that afternoon. The drive home was the longest one I can ever remember.

Which takes us back to earlier advice: You may want to look up the possible side effects of any medication you start taking; ask your pharmacist or doctor if there is anything you should beware of.

Plaquenil also causes sun sensitivity: be sure to wear adequate sunblock and a hat (and long sleeves, if possible) whenever you're out in direct sunlight if you're on an antimalarial medicine. You may not only get sunburned easily, but also develop a rash from where the sun hits your skin.

Finally, Plaquenil can, in rare cases, cause an eye condition known as Plaquenil Retinitis. This form of retinitis shows up to begin with in a field vision test that is performed by your ophthalmologist, which tests your peripheral vision. The bull's-eye pattern of retinitis starts in the outer perimeters of the eyes. Because of this possibility, your doctor will recommend you see an ophthalmologist every six months and have a field vision test performed every six months to one year. If the retinitis starts to present, your doctor will discontinue the Plaquenil

NOTE: Be aware that Advil and other forms of **ibuprofen** are NSAIDs. This means if you have aches and pains, banged your hand while nailing a wall, or have the flu, don't take Advil for those symptoms. You would be possibly doubling your regular dose of NSAIDs that way. Instead, opt for a form of acetaminophen, such as Tylenol, which is a pain reliever but not an NSAID.

immediately. The retinitis won't retreat, but it won't advance, then, either. If caught early enough, you won't experience any loss of vision.

Corticosteroids

These types of steroids are not the kind used by athletes to build muscle tissue—those are metabolic steroids. Instead, **corticosteroids** control inflammatory response by suppressing it, and in conjunction suppress parts of the immune response. Think of corticosteroids working in the same way NSAIDs do, but instead of working against only some of the immune response of inflammation, they work in a more generalized manner against your immune system and inflammation. This is why some doctors and patients refer to corticosteroids as using a "sledgehammer," while NSAIDs are more like using a finishing hammer.

One of the corticosteroids most prescribed is prednisone, which we discussed in some detail in the Living section of this chapter. Another form of corticosteroid is Medrol—which is often dosed out in premeasured packs for a ten-day (or more) course of medication.

The reason Medrol is premeasured in packs stems from the same reason it's so hard to stop taking corticosteroids once a treatment course has begun: You have to slowly increase corticosteroids to achieve their maximum dose; then, when the course is done, you have to slowly decrease the medicine back down to zero. You should not *ever* stop taking corticosteroids cold turkey. The shock to your immune and inflammatory response systems could make you seriously ill. Because you have to ramp up and then back down again, you'll end up staying on the corticosteroids longer than, say, a regular type of short-term medication.

If you have to be on corticosteroids for a long-term period, your doctor will warn you about some of the more serious side effects than simple weight gain; you may experience a decrease in immune response, allowing you to catch communicable illnesses (such as the flu) more easily. In addition, if you do catch a flu or cold, it may worsen more quickly and easily than usual. Heart conditions can also occur.

Corticosteroids are a mixed blessing, bringing both relief from inflammation and illness in lupus, but also allowing more dangerous illnesses to arise. They shouldn't be used casually or for long periods without close supervision of a doctor. After using corticosteroids for a long time, I've done everything I can to stay off of them in order to reduce their side effects, but sometimes it's necessary to take them to save my life.

I have a friend who lost a number of close acquaintances while she was on Medrol: her mood swings, heavy weight gain, and uneven behavior were difficult on everyone. Looking back on it, she refers to it as having PMS (premenstrual syndrome) times ten: she drove everyone crazy, even the ones who knew that it was the medicine she was taking, not anything she could necessarily control at the time.

Chemotherapy

The word *chemotherapy* conjures up scary images for many people, but all it means is a course of chemicals as a means of medicinal therapy. In this case, we're looking at types of chemotherapy administered both orally (by mouth) and intravenously (through an IV drip in a vein) to help curb some of the more serious effects stemming from lupus. By and large, the only people who need to take chemotherapy for lupus are those who have *serious* lupus, which means their organs are affected (such as the lungs, heart, or kidneys). (See Day One for definitions of various types and severities of lupus.)

One drug that constitutes chemotherapy is an immunosuppressant called Imuran. This works by suppressing the body's reaction to stimuli (real or imagined) that would cause the immune system to respond. Because lupus is a disease where the immune system is overreacting, responding to stimuli that don't exist, the condition causes your body to attack perfectly good tissue. Imuran causes the body to repress that response, lowering your immune system to more normal levels. The danger, of course, with any immunosuppressant, is that it can cause you to be more susceptible to communicable diseases that are transmitted from person to person. And once you get ill, you may become more ill than usual—for instance, you may catch the flu, but then it may turn into pneumonia because your body can't fight as easily as usual.

There are a number of immunosuppressants that are administered as chemotherapy on the market today: if you need a course of them, your doctor will talk to you about the pros and cons of taking these kinds of medicine. Some of the common side effects are loss of appetite, weight gain, and sometimes even hair loss.

Antidepressants

Although lupus is not a disease that causes clinical depression through its own merits, it can cause depression because of its effects on your body, your lifestyle, and your mindset. For these reasons, your doctor may prescribe antidepressants for you at some point during your life with lupus.

Another reason why your doctor may explore the use of antidepressants as a medicinal aid in working with your lupus is that it can help with muscle tension while you sleep. Many patients with lupus either have a form of fibromyalgia, restless leg syndrome, or other sleep disturbances caused by muscle tension while they sleep. This causes a great deal of pain and loss of good sleep cycles, often without the patient knowing what the pain and tiredness stems from. Some of the modern antidepressants, such as Prozac, in very small doses, are used

> **NOTE:** Lupus patients should not take supplements that boost the immune system, such as echinacea (purple conehead). Because your immune system is already overactive, you could have a bad reaction to boosting it.

as a nighttime medicine to help the muscles in the body relax sufficiently for deep sleep.

If your doctor prescribes an antidepressant for you, voice your concerns if you think you're being given it for reasons you're not recognizing. Your doctor will assuredly talk to you about the reasons behind his or her thinking, and what the drug is going to do to help your lupus condition.

Vitamins and supplements

A final form of medicine that is considered critical for lupus patients is vitamins, minerals, and other supplements.

Many doctors recommend that lupus patients take a high-dose vitamin B formula multivitamin. Sometimes you can find this packaged as a "women's formula" multivitamin. Vitamin C will help with staving off colds, per some researchers. Trace minerals are also advised, magnesium being one. Check with your doctor as to his or her advice. You can also read up on vitamin research on the Internet; beware of bad research, though. If you read a Web site that's trying to sell you vitamins or supplements, chances are that the research "published" there isn't necessarily scientifically accurate.

Always check with your doctor before adding any vitamins or supplements to your regime.

IN A SENTENCE:

> *Medications are an important part of living a life with lupus, and your doctor will prescribe a range of them as needed for your symptoms and condition.*

Systemic Lupus as a "Women's Disease"

IN DAY One, I briefly touched on the issue of lupus being considered a "women's disease." During week three, we're going to look at this in more depth, particularly the psychosocial aspects of what this is going to mean to you as you live your life with lupus. Whether you're a woman or a man, this issue is going to affect you during your subsequent weeks after diagnosis with the disease, just as it affected you before diagnosis.

Problems of "women's diseases"

Diseases and syndromes that primarily affect women are casually classified as "women's diseases." All this means is that more women than men get these conditions. The problem with this classification is that doctors are taught, both in medical school and through practice in the field, that women—especially in their twenties through forties—often get histrionic illnesses, complaining of many symptoms which don't seem to fit a particular pattern and that change and move rapidly over time.

Many lupus patients run into the problem of doctors assuming that their varying symptoms are "all in the head" or are simple hypochondria, especially in the early stages of the disease presenting itself. This problem is amplified if the patient is a woman, as most developing lupus are in the 20- to 40-year-old range and therefore would fit into the possibly histrionic category. And many lupus patients wonder why it takes so long to get a diagnosis! It can lead to a lot of frustration, anger, and even depression.

Over the years, I have experienced a number of situations where I was treated as if I were a "hysterical" woman, making up symptoms and amplifying nothing into something that surely didn't exist. One particular neurologist actually had the gall to tell me that if I just "dressed nicer" and got out more, I would "get a life" and my imagined illness would go away. Needless to say, I never went to see him again and, in fact, reported the incident to my insurance company. I finally found a wonderful specialist (a gastroenterologist), who was frank with me about how the situation appeared. I already knew that, but was relieved to find someone who would acknowledge that doctors worked that way. I could easily fit that category. He deeply believed I did not—that I did, in fact, have a real disease and real symptoms. Working with him as an adult peer, we explored a number of options, and finally found a good rheumatologist who diagnosed my syndromes and got me on the medications I needed. I still work closely with that gastroenterologist—he literally saved my life.

I hope all lupus patients can find someone as sensitive, thoughtful, and open to working with patients as adults who are in charge of their own lives.

Coping with grief cycles in systemic lupus

Because of this situation, most lupus patients go through grief cycles about their disease. We talked about this during days one through three and again during day seven—this repetition is because grief doesn't just *end*: it cycles throughout your life.

Grief cycles don't all look and act the same way each time you encounter them. In standard grief for a person or loved animal, anniversaries of the death tend to bring the grief cycle around again. For lupus, it's often a flare-up of the disease that brings back all the anger, frustration, and grief again. This means you're going to cycle through all those feelings over and over again in what is often termed "complicated grief."

Complicated grief is the type that doesn't end its cycles in a regular fashion and/or is triggered more often than a simple anniversary. So in a way, all lupus patients can experience complicated grief during their lives. This is *normal* for anybody with a chronic disease or condition. A good friend of mine has become a quadriplegic after being quite active all of his life. Michael cycles through complicated grief in the same way a lupus patient does—so do people with multiple sclerosis or epilepsy or fibromyalgia. The feelings all these people go through are very normal, though not very pleasant for the patients themselves.

Treatment for complicated grief in the chronically ill can take a few forms, but one is, of course, medication with antidepressants. Most lupus patients take a mild dose of antidepressants for pain relief at night, which can also act as a psychotropic dose. If you feel as if you need help with your grief, anger, or depression about having lupus, talk to your doctor—there are antidepressants on the market that have reasonably mild side effects and are very effective in treating this type of depression. Talk therapy is also useful. Remember your support group? That's part of what they're there for: to listen to you and let you vent about how it sucks to have this disease. Groups of lupus patients often meet at local clinics, hospitals, and even bookstore/cafes to talk to each other about living with lupus. Give a call to your local hospital and see if they know of any groups in your area. Sometimes nothing beats talking to someone who knows *exactly* what you're going through.

Get out of the house!

I can't emphasize enough the importance of social interaction when you have lupus. It's so easy to wallow in your own pain and grief, especially when you're in a flare. Getting out and meeting with other people is very important when you have a chronic disease, in large part because you need to get out of your own head, so to speak. It's easy to fall into a cycle of grief and pain if you don't have the distraction of interacting with others, even if it's just to go to a movie or out for a cup of coffee.

I work at home, which is a situation many lupus patients end up creating for themselves, mostly to reduce stress. Stresswise, it's fantastic to work at home, but socially it's very isolating. A few years ago I made a vow to myself that I'd get out of the house and go have lunch at a local restaurant at least once a week, socialize with some people that go there for their lunch breaks, and get in some good conversation that had (1) nothing to do with my work, and (2) had nothing to do with having lupus. It's been wonderful, and I've made some good friends that way.

Even if you don't work at home, make sure you have social time with others that don't necessarily have lupus or another chronic disease. Or if they do, you may want to try to have a book talk or a movie night or a coffee klatch that has nothing to do with talking about your illnesses: get out of your own world of chronic illness for a few hours, and you'll see a change in your stress levels, too.

Educating others

As we discussed earlier in this chapter, doctors often have a negative reaction to women who have a wide range of symptoms and conditions, even if they are already diagnosed with a chronic disease such as lupus. I've seen it firsthand in one primary care physician I had, who wanted "nothing to do with lupus-anything"—in other words, unless I had a broken leg or a hangnail, she wanted nothing to do with my medical treatment. She wanted only the rheumatologist to treat anything that I came down with, including simple pneumonia. Why? She apparently felt overwhelmed with the idea of a patient who had a tide of symptoms and conditions that she would have to treat, and so started to think of me as a "difficult woman." Women's diseases, again.

The general public often feels the same way doctors do; even our own friends and family may feel something akin to this. It's our job to educate them as we can, allowing them to learn that lupus is a disease that comes and goes with flares, can manifest in many ways and with many conditions and illnesses, and that we're not just "making it up."

When you have lupus, you usually don't *look* sick. That's a problem. We're chronically ill, and yet we don't necessarily have a limp, we don't have obvious medical anomalies showing, we don't talk funny or look funny. And yet we're *ill*. It's hard to get people to understand that we're not going to ever be completely well again—unless we go into full remission (which isn't outside the realm of possibility). But for most of us, we're going to have flares and good times, ebbing and flowing, the rest of our lives.

People expect us to "buck up" and "act like we look." We're expected, as a friend of mine wrote in her book, *Making Book,* to learn to play the piano with our noses. I couldn't ever say it better than she has. Teresa Nielsen Hayden has a rare form of narcolepsy, and wrote this essay while she was trying to relearn how to write again after discovering what it's like to live with a chronic illness that isn't evident to the naked eye:

16. New York (no date): Spitting in the Ocean, Railing at Fate.

Once upon a time . . . once upon a time I was twenty years old and made the Dean's List while holding down three part-time jobs and taking regular instruction at the local Newman Center (I'd decided that I would never understand medieval literature without understanding Catholicism), plus pursuing an expansive and cheerfully peculiar social life. Hardly anyone I know anymore remembers me from that time, long ago, far away, no acquaintances in common et cetera. Fewer remember what I was like back in high school.

I grieve myself with the suspicion that people who meet me these days think I'm naturally slow-moving, indolent, easily confused, erratic, quicker to modify and mollify than to argue straight out. And that hurts, it makes me want to yell something like "I wasn't always like this! I'm not a happy underachiever! I—"

They have no reason to believe me. Who could? I think the only relic left from those days is a certain ungodly prickliness: chin up, a direct stare, and who the hell do you think you are?—as if it were still perfectly self-evident (to me) that the person I address is, if well-meaning, still intolerably presumptuous.

A quick test, two famous lines: which come more trippingly off the tongue?

"I have always depended on the kindness of strangers."

"Are *you* talking to *me*?"

It has its uses, for which I suppose I should be grateful; but when your chief remaining stock in trade is unwarranted arrogance, a much-mended and lovingly repolished assumption of ability that glosses over any number of small inexplicable errors or failures of memory—the audience sometimes buys it, and I pretend I do—dwelling upon the Sunday-school virtue of humble gratitude for whatever mites you still possess can seem dangerous.

I despise articles (they're usually in *Reader's Digest*) about saintly, courageous, forbearing cripples and invalids who, against all odds, succeed in not only surviving, but in learning to play the piano with their nose. Or something just as arbitrary, like parachuting into a national park or getting a job. Yes, it's true—born tragically deformed, entirely lacking a skeleton, little Marina nonetheless persevered and today works half-days as a beautician! And it only took thirty-four years for her to reach that goal! O Triumph for the Challenged, oh barf. (Way to go, Marina. *You* I'll applaud.)

Healthy people wouldn't work for years, with unflagging determination, to be able to do that. The deed itself is not the point. The mastery is, the sense of having some control over your own life, of making a satisfactory accommodation. Which can be heroic (not me, I'm whining for all I'm worth), but is nothing you'd *choose* to do.

Okay, so I feel guilty riffing about this. I have almost all my original body parts, in recognizable condition. I'm not in constant pain, and, God willing, I'm not likely to die this year. I even have partial medical coverage. So maybe I don't have much room to complain, except when the people who tell me so are much healthier than I am and don't seem to judge the success and happiness of their own lives by comparing them to a quadriplegic's, any more than the ones who point out that my life is better than that of most Third-Worlders would be pleased if I served them a dinner of grasshoppers, manioc, and edible weeds.

I don't know. Maybe I'm being a jerk about this; I genuinely can't tell. But if I am, I apologize. Honest.

It's just that those stories strike me as ghost-repellent. You know, ghosts like in *Macbeth,* the part where Banquo wanders into the banquet looking ectoplasmic and ghastly, and says, "The race is neither to the swift, nor the contest to the one with the hot SAT scores; all the promise your grandmother was sure you showed guarantees you exactly nothing, even if by some chance she was right, and in a pinch even hard work and determination won't necessarily prevail (though I must admit, Lady Macbeth, they help; my compliments, after a fashion). We're all hostages to chance, temporarily able-bodied, temporarily young, temporarily capable."

This is something nobody wants to hear, that the profit a man hath for all the labour he taketh under the sun amounts to a lottery ticket, time of drawing uncertain. Not Macbeth, that's for sure; under the spectre's gaze he gets red in the face, chokes as he tries to clear his throat—then watches in complete dumb incomprehension as Banquo suddenly totters a bit, blinks rapidly, and collapses, snoring, into a handy chair. No telling how soon he'll wake up, either, and in the meantime his half-slumped, half-sprawled form is a graceless singularity amidst the festive scene. The guests all leave; the Macbeths, deeply irritated, retire for the evening. When Banquo wakes up he finds himself in an empty, disorderly hall, tables still strewn with the fragments and remnants of someone else's party. He wanders around disconsolately, eats a couple of cold chicken wings, and departs.

The nicest, kindest people in the world can turn out to feel an . . . intolerable discomfort . . . around serious illness, injury, disability, if they've never had their own chops smitten with a comparable lightning bolt. Dear friend, do you want to bet it can't happen to you? Of course it can, and you know it. Those who eat nothing but kelp and wheat germ and trail mix, and regularly irrigate their chakras and immune systems, who can talk for hours about the correct mental attitudes to prevent arthritis and cancer, are paying homage to that chance. So are the ones who boast that they stay up 'til all hours smoking cigarettes and listening to low-fidelity jazz recordings, who eat only Reese's Peanut Butter Cups and taco-flavored nacho chips: why else go to that much trouble to moon Fate? And it can happen anytime—lumps in the flesh, strange effusions, open gas-flame water heaters, foot-pounds per second, chemistries gone subtly awry.

Terrible! You? Not you, no. Hey, it's cool. I didn't think it would happen to me, either, you know? Except that it's been a while now, and it gets less all right with me all the time. You get the news—the horror, the horror—but at least it's an answer. It's a novelty. Then it isn't a novelty at all, but it's just as much trouble as ever. The realization starts to sink in: You're never going to get to quit thinking about this. You start to appreciate the finer points of its irritations; sore points get rubbed raw. And Christ it's boring.

That's the other thing about Inspirational Crip stories: they leave out the dreary bits, the times when heroic effort is what it takes to wash the breakfast dishes. I know they're fake because they never, ever let on that being sick all the time is boring. Boring, boring, boring. Really boring. Then, just when you think you can't stand it anymore, it gets boring for a while. And once in a while something terrifying happens; just to keep you on your toes. Then it goes back to being boring. And you find yourself thinking, "Maybe I could learn to play the piano with my nose. Anything's better than this."

(Teresa Nielsen Hayden, *Making Book*. NESFA Press, 1996. Used with permission.)

IN A SENTENCE:

> *Because lupus is considered a "women's disease," it's important to acknowledge the complicated grief that problem will cause, and seek out support from others, including educating others as to lupus's chronic condition.*

learning

Historical & Modern Expectations and Prognosis of Lupus

HISTORICAL VERSUS modern prognoses of lupus are like night and day. The entire outlook on lupus has changed significantly in the last ten years; even twenty years ago, most lupus patients died quickly after diagnosis. Why? Because diagnosis was usually made far too late for anything to be done for fatal conditions such as terminal kidney failure. With the advance of a blood test for the ANA factor, showing rheumatoid conditions in the body, and the list of lupus symptoms we went over in day one, diagnosis is now made much more quickly and effectively than ever before.

Even though no one still knows for certain what causes lupus, doctors can treat a patient much faster and with greater accuracy, leading to lupus now being considered a chronic but not necessarily fatal disease. Most lupus patients don't die of lupus, per se, but usually something completely unrelated, or by an illness brought on by a depressed immune system from taking immunosuppressants such as chemotherapy (see Week Two: Learning).

Early diagnosis is important

Seeking out a diagnosis is critically important. And it's sometimes very difficult, as you already know. My own search for a diagnosis took over a decade and more frustration than I want to remember, but it was ultimately worth it: effective treatment. Without good treatment, a lupus patient is putting her- or himself in danger of medical difficulties. Lupus flares can range from tendonitis to pericarditis (inflammation of the sac surrounding the heart), and without diagnosis and therefore proper treatment, the lupus sufferer could be in a lot of trouble down the line.

One famous actress, Kelly Martin (starred in *ER*), had a sister with lupus. Unfortunately her sister wasn't diagnosed for any number of years, despite the family's efforts to get doctors to define her disease and treat it. By the time she was diagnosed, her lupus had progressed to her organs and severely affected her overall health; she died within a year of diagnosis.

This grim story isn't what happens to everyone, but it is what used to happen before effective diagnostic techniques for lupus were available. And it still happens to people who don't actively seek out diagnosis and aren't diligent about finding a doctor who will find an answer to their symptoms. Even with active work to find a diagnostician who can recognize complicated lupus, sometimes people—like Kelly Martin's sister—fall through the cracks.

Lupus is difficult to diagnose sometimes. There's no question about it. But the onus often falls on us, the patients, to push our doctors to find an answer. Sometimes the answer is finding another doctor, or even travelling to find a specialty diagnostician, such as those found at the Lahey Clinic. Whatever the means, I can't emphasize enough that it's important for you to find some sort of effective treatment for your condition, and that usually means a diagnosis of lupus or one of its related syndromes (see Month Two). Do what you have to do to find out what's up with your health.

Educating Doctors

Finally, we need to work as a group and individually to educate doctors and other health workers about lupus and how it is indeed a "women's disease" but is not necessarily part of the "difficult woman's syndrome." You know what I mean: the woman who complains about the aches and pains and this and that and usually it's because she's bored and has nothing to do with her life. She goes from doctor to doctor, annoying one after the other, and no diagnosis is ever made because there's nothing actually wrong with her. We've probably all been treated as if we're that woman, at one point or another. Why? Because, as I said earlier, doctors are educated to recognize "women's diseases" as being equivalent to the "difficult woman syndrome."

But they're not the same. Lupus is a disease primarily affecting women, but it's a valid, chronic, rheumatological disease that affects the immune system. Just because we approach doctors with a multitude of symptoms—some of which appear and disappear rapidly—doesn't mean we aren't actually chronically ill. Proper diagnosis of lupus usually ends the attitude doctors have toward us as "difficult" women, but sometimes it continues because of an unconscious diagnosis they've already made that we're "complainers."

The same group of changing symptoms, when presented by a man rather than a woman, usually provokes a different response. Men aren't usually typified as complainers, even if they present exactly the same as women. Doctors need to learn to treat women the same as men, especially during the diagnostic stage of treatment—and this may only change if we demand this sort of equality.

IN A SENTENCE:

Historically lupus has been a dangerous disease, but no longer through fast and effective diagnosis, though work is still needed to educate doctors in diagnosing women without treating them as though they are being histrionic.

"I Feel Like I've Lost My Mind"

LUPUS HAS neurological and psychological effects that are accounted for by most patients but are mostly undocumented scientifically by the medical community. During week four, we'll take a look at some of those effects, how to deal with them, coping techniques, as well as what cerebral lupus (CNS) is and how it is treated.

"Lupus fog"

Remember how in Days Six and Seven I mentioned a "fog" that can come over lupus and fibromyalgia patients? That fog is for real—it's a neurological effect of lupus that is reported by most people who have the disease. It seems to come and go, usually getting worse during flares.

Lupus fog has many symptoms, including:

- forgetfulness
- loss of short-term memory
- aphasia or loss of words

- clumsiness
- fatigue
- inability to multitask
- distractedness

During a lupus fog, you will feel as if someone pulled the rug out from under you. Recall Teresa Nielsen Hayden's essay at the end of the Living section of Week Three, in which she sums up the feeling of having lost her ability to be brilliant, graceful, and strong:

> I grieve myself with the suspicion that people who meet me these days think I'm naturally slow-moving, indolent, easily confused, erratic, quicker to modify and mollify than to argue straight out. And that hurts, it makes me want to yell something like "I wasn't always like this! I'm not a happy underachiever! I—" (used with permission from *Making Book*, Teresa Nielsen Hayden)

Most people with lupus can associate with these words immediately —lupus fog makes you feel as if you've lost your mind. Memory loss is difficult for anyone, but for someone who also has chronic conditions stemming from lupus, it makes it doubly hard. Your body seems to be working against you, and now your mind isn't cooperating, either.

Coping with lupus fog & memory loss

What to do? Coping behaviors can help you deal with everyday life a little bit better. People may not notice your memory loss periods during lupus fog if you learn a few "tricks" to cover your flare. I'm not advocating that you ignore your symptoms from the fog—if you have serious memory loss that causes you to forget common things such as your name or your spouse's hair color, you need to talk to your doctor immediately.

- Have someone go with you to medical appointments and the like—your memory person, sort of like a seeing-eye dog.

I refer to my husband, Andrew, as my "memo pad," since he remembers things for me when I'm in a fog. I'm lucky that way. You may need to pick someone from your support group to do the same thing for you. If you're alone and don't have someone to help out with passing memory problems, try a small tape recorder or a Palm Pilot (or other PDA); record or write down the smallest, most trivial items, when you're in a fog. That way when the fog tries to delete them from your short-term memory, you'll always have the information somewhere you can remember. I call my Palm my "brain"—it is, indeed, my external brain. I'd be lost without it.

(NOTE: If you do rely on a PDA or a tape recorder to help with short-term memory, *back up the information somewhere*. Always have a second copy! Mechanical objects eventually fail, and you could lose precious information forever.)

○   Make a list of important information, such as your telephone number, your support person's daytime phone number, your doctor's phone number, and a list of your medications.

Put it in a place you can always find it, such as the front of your refrigerator. Repeat to yourself, as you put that list up, that you *can always find the list there.* Go to the list frequently, so you embed in your long-term memory that it's there.

If you have major memory slippage, you can then go to the list and call either your support person or your doctor. If something happens and emergency personnel come to your house, your list of medications will also be there.

Over time, you will develop generalized coping techniques to get you through lupus fog. No one person can tell you how you're going to react to memory slippage, increased clumsiness, etc. Only you can and will develop little tricks to get you through your fog times—hang in there, you will learn them! I have some dear friends who know how I can get and joke about it; I joke back with them about my IQ slipping or about how I used to be a ballet dancer (I was!). Sometimes the jokes

> **NOTE:** You should make what is called a Vial of L.I.F.E. (Lifesaving Informa-
> tion For Emergencies). You will put a list of your medications in a large, old,
> empty pill bottle (amber in color) on the top shelf of your refrigerator in the
> front. You can get a form for the vial at any local fire department, or download
> it in Acrobat format here: http://www.sjfd.com/Vial_of_Life.pdf. If emergency
> medical services have to come to your house, they are trained to first look in
> your fridge for that vial of information about your medicines.

help—it makes me feel like a normal person. Other times, with strangers, I cover my memory lapses with long pauses in my conversation as if I always talked slowly and deliberately, as if I were thinking hard about what the other person was just saying. Sometimes it works; sometimes I come off as being a ditzy lady. Either way, I have learned to not mind it too much—those people who know me and love me know it's just lupus fog, and that I'm just as smart as I ever was. It's just that sometimes it goes behind a fogbank for a few days at a time!

Personality effects and changes

You will change in many ways from having lupus. Being chronically ill changes a person forever, and there's nothing you can do about that. What you need to concentrate on is the *positive* changes you can effect in your life.

Memory loss and fog are going to change how you interact with others, even those close to you. Your personality will, to a degree, change and modify itself to account for your changes in memory and daily interactions. You won't be the same person you were before.

The trick is being a person you want to be, a person you would like to be. The gaps in memory, the changes in the way you think and move and live, these are all going to make you a new person in some ways. You will want to shift your gaze to focusing on how you can take your energies and create changes that are positive rather than negative. Sure, you forget where your car keys are most of the time, but does that make you into a grumpy person who swears like a sailor every time she misplaces her keys? Instead, you may want to be the person who laughs and makes a game out of finding her keys. Or, better yet, a person who says, "What can I do to help myself not forget my keys?" And then goes out and buys one of those key rings that beeps back at you when you call to it or clap your hands. Then the keys are rarely lost—they're only a handclap away.

Be inventive. Ask your support group, whether friends/family or fellow lupus patients, for suggestions on how you can help cope with lupus fog and still stay positive and keep a personality that others want to be around. No one wants to be around a grumpy, swearing, feel-sorry-for-yourself sort of person—not for very long.

I know I sound like Pollyana again, but it's all quite true. I'm not perfect; I forget things and get angry and stomp around and go sulk and feel sorry for myself at least once in a while (okay, more than once in a while!), but I continue to work at knowing that, compared to many people, I'm lucky. I'm not going to necessarily die of this disease, and a bit of lupus fog and memory slippage comes with the territory. And I pick myself up, make jokes, and go on. You can learn to do the same—you'll learn how *you* cope and create a new lifestyle around that.

IN A SENTENCE:

Lupus fog can cause you to have some memory loss side effects, but you can learn to cope with them and create a lifestyle that's positive.

learning

A Clinical Approach to Neurological Effects of Lupus

LUPUS HAS effects on the mind as well as being able to have physical effects on the brain itself, though that's a rarity. There are clinical approaches to diagnosing these effects, as well as coping techniques that can be applied through medicinal and other therapeutic programs.

Although there is no "cure" for the mind fog and memory losses brought on by lupus, there are therapies that can help with the effects. Lupus fog is known clinically as **cognitive dysfunction**. Two primary treatments are the use of drugs and psychological therapies. In addition to lupus fog there are several other neurological effects, including lupus headache, peripheral neuropathy, and central nervous system (CNS) vasculitis.

• • •

Cognitive dysfunction

Lupus fog is termed cognitive dysfunction by physicians. It manifests as confusion, forgetfulness, memory loss, inability to express thoughts, and fatigue. It is, in essence, almost indistinguishable from the "fibro fog" shown in fibromyalgia patients. No one knows for certain what causes it, but it is widely assumed to stem from inflammation in the blood vessels that flow to the brain and central nervous system, or inflammation in the nerve bundles themselves. The effects of cognitive dysfunction can, in fact, be measured using equipment such as an MRI (magnetic resonance imager) machine in a hospital—it will show decreased blood flow to certain parts of the brain during a session of cognitive dysfunction.

Two methods are often used to combat cognitive dysfunction: drug therapy, and psychotherapy or counseling.

DRUG THERAPY

As we discussed in Day Seven, certain drugs seem to help with alleviating clinical chronic fatigue. Those same drugs seem to help to a degree with the effects of mind fog and some of its presentations, such as fatigue, "ditziness," distractedness, and an inability to multitask. Some memory problems don't seem to be relieved by these drugs, but some people react very positively to them overall for the fog effects. The primary medicines used for this are antidepressants, especially the newer varieties, such as Prozac or Effexor. Another one that seems to help with the fatigue is Plaquenil, an antimalarial drug. Sometimes corticosteroids are used to combat fatigue. Your doctor will determine what might be the best medicine for you to try to help with your fog symptoms.

One of the problems you may encounter when talking to your doctor about these symptoms is getting her or him to believe that it's not just simply depression. After all, you're chronically ill, and doctors are taught that chronically ill people are naturally depressed. Talk to your physician about what constitutes lupus fog. If you are having a problem talking about it effectively, your rheumatologist may be more under-standing, since they're trained specifically in lupus conditions. If push comes to shove, take in some information from the Lupus Foundation of America for them to read. You can download some information on lupus fog from their Web site: http://www.lupus.org. They also have brochures and books available from their bookstore. Call: 301-670-9292 (Rockville, MD).

Friends of mine on the lupus mailing list to which I belong often bemoan their doctors disbelieving, or underemphasizing, any cognitive dysfunction they report. It's a theme I've heard from other lupus patients for almost a decade: "My doctor's not listening to me" or "My doctor is treating me like I'm an idiot" or even "My doctor is treating me like I'm simply crazy." It's a difficult situation, since you may actually *become* depressed from having your symptoms downplayed or even ignored by your physician. Take heart: you're not the only one who has this happen. What can you do about it? Read on.

Remember, depression is also normal for the lupus patient. It's part and parcel of being chronically ill, in pain, suffering fatigue and mem-ory problems, and sometimes by necessity being cut off from people because you are sick and need to rest often. If your doctor suspects you're depressed, this isn't the end of the world. You're not a failure. Depression is a clinical illness, just like your lupus—most researchers think it's caused by a lack of certain neurotransmitters firing correctly in the brain. Antidepressants help rebalance this loss, and that's why you'll end up feeling better. Don't be afraid to talk to your physician about any questions or misgivings you have about your depression and taking antidepressants—that's what your doctor is there for.

PSYCHOLOGICAL THERAPIES

Your doctor also might want you to see a psychologist, psychiatrist, or clinical social worker for some therapy. There are types of talk and behavioral therapies that can help with the effects of lupus fog and memory problems. This will probably be in conjunction with a course of antidepressants—it's usually recommended that therapy always accompany these types of medicines, as they go hand in hand in order to help you adjust your lifestyle.

Your therapist can help be your support through some of the problems and questions you're going to have when you have lupus fog: memory loss, fatigue, clumsiness—all of those effects we talked about in the Living section, above. Remember how I talked about bringing your life into a positive stance, no matter that you were going to change as a person because of the lupus fog and other effects on your mind and personality? Your therapist can help with this, too.

If possible, find a therapist who has dealt with lupus patients before. If not, you may be able to more easily find one who's dealt with fibromyalgia patients—they go through very similar effects from what's called "fibro fog." You should be able to learn some positive coping techniques as well as lifestyle changes you can make in order to learn to live more fully with your lupus, fog and all.

Lupus headaches

Lupus headaches manifest as anything from severe tension headaches to migraines. Your doctor will probably send you to a neurologist for diagnosis, to determine what sort of headache you're getting, and to make sure it's actually emanating from lupus or being caused by another condition.

One lupus friend I have has such bad headaches she is on high-dose migraine medications for it, so high she's had side effects from them such as hand tremors. The side effects, however, are nothing compared to a migraine that keeps her on the couch in a dark room until (or if) it subsides. Some of her migraines are so bad she can't stand up and can't hold a conversation while one is ongoing. You can only imagine what this does to her work schedule.

Many lupus patients don't realize that their headaches are related to lupus until a rheumatologist or neurologist tells them so. If you're encountering bad headaches, talk to your physician about a referral to a neurologist; it may be that he or she can help you sort out if you're having a "lupus headache," and if it can be helped with medication they can prescribe.

Lupus headaches are treated with regular migraine medication or corticosteroids, which are usually effective.

Peripheral neuropathy

Peripheral neuropathy simply means that you have nerve dysfunction in any part of your body other than your brain or spinal cord. It usually occurs in a limb—arm or leg—or fingers or toes.

You could have tingling, burning, or itching sensations. Many lupus patients report an itching feeling, as if they have a rash, but no rash is present. This can be quite disconcerting if you don't know that this is a "normal" symptom for a lupus patient. Do not, however, ignore any loss of sensation or tingling you may have: get it checked out by a doctor. After all, it could be caused by any number of things, such as a pinched nerve or even a small stroke (blood clot in the brain). Your physician can determine if the neuropathy you're experiencing is caused by the lupus or by another condition.

Again, corticosteroids are usually used to treat peripheral neuropathy, but your doctor may also have other suggestions.

Central Nervous System (CNS) lupus

CNS lupus is one of the severe variations of the disease, and when it manifests must be treated immediately by your doctor, usually in a hospital setting.

CNS lupus happens when the the blood vessels that feed your brain become inflamed—this condition is known as **vasculitis**. Symptoms of CNS lupus include:

○ seizures
○ confusion
○ high fever

○ stiff neck (acting like meningitis)

○ psychosis

High doses of corticosteroids are administered to a CNS lupus patient; if seizures occur, you might also be given anticonvulsant medicines to control them. Note that these seizures will probably not come back once the vasculitis is under control.

Interestingly, CNS vasculitis is the only central nervous system condition recognized as being part of lupus by the American College of Rheumatology's criteria for diagnosing lupus.

Only ten percent of lupus patients ever experience CNS vasculitis, so there's only a small chance this will happen to you. If it does, your doctor will hospitalize you and get it under control; it may never reoccur.

IN A SENTENCE:

> *Neurological effects of lupus include cognitive dysfunction, lupus headache, peripheral neuropathy, and central nervous system (CNS) vasculitis.*

FIRST-MONTH MILESTONE

By the end of your first month, you have armed yourself with more knowledge about lupus and its effects on your life and the lives of those around you.

You have learned:

○ WHICH DRUGS ARE USED FOR LUPUS TREATMENT.

○ HOW TO ORGANIZE YOUR MEDICATIONS.

○ WHY LUPUS IS CONSIDERED A "WOMEN'S DISEASE."

○ HOW TO COPE WITH ONGOING GRIEF CYCLES.

○ HOW TO EDUCATE OTHERS ABOUT YOUR DISEASE, EVEN IF IT'S SOMETIMES "INVISIBLE."

○ COGNITIVE DYSFUNCTION IN LUPUS (THE "LUPUS FOG").

Overlapping Syndromes

As I mentioned in Day One, lupus doesn't occur in a vacuum. Most of the time, it shows up with overlapping syndromes and conditions. This is called overlapping lupus. Chances are, you have, or will develop during your lifetime, at least one overlapping syndrome. These syndromes include fibromyalgia, the lupus "mask," Sjögren's Syndrome, Raynaud's Syndrome, and a variety of conditions that can affect your heart, lungs, blood, digestion, and kidneys.

Living with overlapping lupus

It's not easy to live with a disease that can pop up with a new condition at any moment. It's also not easy living with a disease that can suddenly develop sister or brother syndromes without warning. But that's how lupus works, for good or ill. What's important is learning how to cope with the consequences.

It's possibly going to be an overwhelming feeling the first time your rheumatologist or primary care physician says that he or she thinks you may have another syndrome that often is carried with lupus. After all, you thought you were done with diagnoses and you were on the road to living with your disease, knowing all the things that could possibly happen to you. Instead, now you're being told you have *another* illness, another condition with its own quirks and symptoms, to deal with.

Don't feel overwhelmed. It's unusual *not* to have an overlapping syndrome. Most people with lupus have at least one additional syndrome or chronic condition to handle. Since most syndromes that get carried with lupus are treated in a similar manner to lupus itself, it's possible you won't need many new medications or lifestyle changes. What you will need is some education as to what your syndrome can do to you. We'll discuss those in more detail in the following months, as we go through several syndromes one at a time in detail.

For now know that you're not alone, and the same support groups that can be found for lupus patients exist for people with syndromes such as Sjögren's and Raynaud's.

Helping other people understand

You will need to take some time and effort to help educate the people around you about these additional syndromes. After all, they've already had to learn to deal with your lupus symptoms, and now there will be more.

I've found, after I was diagnosed with both Sjögren's and Raynaud's syndromes, that having multiple symptoms, which come and go (sometimes depending on the weather or season, or stress levels), all erratically, causes a negative reaction in most of the people around you. After all, most people who display that sort of health pattern are usually hypochondriacs. It can be frustrating to deal with people who clearly think "it's all in your head," especially when you "suddenly" start showing a whole new set of symptoms. The worst frustration comes for people who previously seemed to finally understand how a life with lupus would affect your relationship with them, and now, when you display a new syndrome, they don't understand your lifestyle and health issues—all over again.

We're back to educating the people around us. The next chapters should help you explain some of the syndromes you may develop. No matter what the syndrome or condition, however, education of the people around you is going to be the primary means of having them learn to cope with your condition. They'll need to learn to make compromises —you will too!—yet again. They'll need to learn when and how to push you to be more positive, and when to let you cry and vent your frustration. And they'll need to learn what conditions—such as stress, or exposure to sunlight—will make your new syndrome(s) flare up and get worse.

Diagnosis of overlapping syndromes

Now that we've put the cart before the horse, let's cast back to the diagnosis of your new overlapping syndrome(s). You will probably have displayed some sort of new symptoms, or had your previous symptoms suddenly take on a pattern that your physician now recognizes, and you'll have been recommended to either go see your rheumatologist or even yet another specialist.

Your specialist will do a number of tests, depending on what syndrome he or she thinks you may have. We'll go over those in more detail in the following months. For now, you need to concentrate on what your specialist is seeing in all these symptoms. Hopefully they are following an obvious pattern and your diagnosis will be an easy, quick one. Unfortunately, just as with lupus, it's probable that your symptoms may be a bit of a jumble and hard to decipher.

If you are female and have a mountain of seemingly patternless symptoms, your physician may start looking at you as if you're one of those "difficult women." Remember how we talked about that attitude during Week Three (Learning section)? This is going to be another time when you may have to confront your doctor about how he or she is treating you differently than if you were a man with the same symptoms. You're going to need to tread carefully, but you should be able to explain your symptoms in a systematic manner—write them down in a list before you go in to see the doctor. Let the doctor know that you know that this appears to be like a "difficult woman" sort of situation, but you honestly feel that because you are already diagnosed with lupus, you probably are displaying some sort of overlapping syndrome or condition. Then ask your doctor if he or she can help you figure out why you're having new symptoms. Let her know that you *want* to feel better, that you don't *like* being sick.

To reiterate, if you feel as if you are getting nowhere with your physician and feel as if your health is being threatened due to lack of treatment, ask to see if you or they can provide a patient advocate. If that doesn't help, you need to make the hard consideration of finding a new doctor. I've seen and spoken to far too many lupus patients who end up critically ill because their doctors ignored their symptoms from overlapping syndromes, treating them as if they were "difficult women." Some are now permanently disabled from their conditions; if they had gotten adequate diagnostic care and treatment in good time, they would be living with their lupus far more comfortably to this day.

Remember: You are your best advocate. Be firm, when you need to be, about receiving adequate medical care.

IN A SENTENCE:

> *Most lupus patients develop overlapping syndromes, which can often make it difficult—all over again—for people, including doctors, to understand what it's like to live with lupus.*

learning

Common Overlapping Syndromes with Lupus

THERE ARE several overlapping syndromes that occur often with systemic lupus. These include:

○ Sjögren's Syndrome
○ Raynaud's Syndrome
○ fibromyalgia
○ the lupus "mask"
○ various conditions with the body's systems
  ○ pulmonary
  ○ circulatory
  ○ digestive
  ○ kidney

Sjögren's Syndrome

This syndrome comes in two varieties: Primary Sjögren's and Secondary Sjögren's. The first occurs by itself, and the second is usually an overlapping syndrome with lupus. The syndrome is named for the doctor who first recognized it as a medical condition.

Both varieties of Sjögren's manifest in just about the same way; the only real difference is that secondary Sjögren's doesn't usually affect the organs of the body, as primary can. Both varieties act just like lupus, in that they are rheumatological, autoimmune syndromes where the body is attacking perfectly good tissue by being hyperactive. But in the case of Sjögren's, it primarily attacks the connective tissues of the body responsible for creating mucus, which includes the tear ducts, salivary glands, ducts in the digestive tract, and, in the case of women, in the vaginal area. What happens is the body fails to make enough fluid and you get very dry. This can be anything from painful to dangerous to your health.

There are a number of effective treatments for Sjögren's, which we'll discuss in a chapter about this syndrome during Month Three.

Raynaud's Syndrome

This syndrome occurs when the body attacks the circulatory system in the peripheral parts of your body (fingers and toes), again as if it were a foreign agent and the autoimmune system had to fight it off. Raynaud's is another of the rheumatological, autoimmune syndromes.

When you have Raynaud's, your fingers and toes will get extremely cold or even burning hot, but no temperature change is evident in the rest of the hand or foot. The fingers or toes will turn bright red or pale white. During the winter, care must be taken by the Raynaud's patient to make sure fingers and toes aren't exposed to extreme temperature changes, or damage to the tissue can result.

Raynaud's is usually categorized as part of discoid, or skin, lupus, since it affects the circulatory system and the epidermis. There are treatments for Raynaud's that we will explore more during Month Three.

The lupus "mask"

The infamous wolflike "mask" of lupus is really the malar rash that occurs for some lupus patients and primarily in people who have discoid, or skin, lupus. It is usually a red, sometimes brownish, mask-like pattern in a butterfly shape over the nose and across the cheeks. it doesn't itch or burn like most rashes, but it does come and go, usually depending on a flare-up of your condition.

A picture of the lupus mask can be found in Month Four.

Secondary conditions to lupus

There are several conditions secondary to lupus that can occur. These include alterations to the following body systems: pulmonary, circulatory, digestive, and the kidneys. We'll talk about these conditions in more detail in the months that follow. For now, let's take a quick look at each as an overview.

PULMONARY

Your pulmonary system includes your lungs and the lining around them, which is called the pleural lining. One of the common conditions that lupus patients can get is pleurisy, which is an inflammation of the lining surrounding the lungs. That lining can also fill with fluid; when that happens, it's called a pleural effusion.

CIRCULATORY

Some lupus patients are prone to developing blood clots (deep vein thrombosis, or **DVT**), and some show what is called the **lupus anti-coagulant factor** (antiphospholipid antibody) in their blood. Both cause conditions in the blood to either make it clot more easily or make it harder for it to clot, and therefore easier to bleed freely. People who have Raynaud's Syndrome and/or Sjögren's Syndrome tend to get blood clots more easily.

DIGESTIVE

A number of people with lupus seem to develop digestive issues, particularly if they also have fibromyalgia. **Irritable Bowel Syndrome (IBS)** and other irritations and inflammations of the bowel, which come and go with flares, are not uncommon.

KIDNEYS & LIVER

For those lupus patients who are on long-term use of particular drugs such as immunosuppressants and NSAIDs (like Celebrex), effects on the kidneys can sometimes occur. Your doctor will monitor your kidney and liver functions carefully whenever you're taking a medication that puts extra work on those organs. In some rare cases, lupus patients develop kidney failure—this used to be more common when lupus went undiagnosed for many years, but is less common nowadays.

IN A SENTENCE:

> *Common syndromes that can be seen overlapping with lupus are: Sjögren's Syndrome, Raynaud's Syndrome, fibromyalgia, the lupus mask, and conditions that affect the pulmonary, circulatory, digestive, and kidney functions of the body.*

learning

Sjögren's and Raynaud's Syndromes

AS WE briefly discussed in the previous month, there are two major syndromes that are often carried along with lupus: Sjögren's and Raynaud's Syndromes. Both are named for the physicians who first categorized them as specific rheumatological conditions.

What is Sjögren's Syndrome?

Sjögren's is a rheumatological syndrome that manifests in two manners. Primary Sjögren's appears by itself, while secondary Sjögren's shows up along with another rheumatological disease, usually lupus. The syndrome primarily affects the tear ducts, salivary glands, and other mucal glands in places such as the digestive tract and—in women—the vagina. However, it can also affect most of the connective tissues of the body, similar to lupus. Primary Sjögren's will be present with symptoms almost identical to lupus in many ways, while secondary Sjögren's only shows up in the mucal glands.

Primary Sjögren's symptoms include (in brief):

- dry eyes
- dry mouth
- digestive anomalies
- pleurisy
- pericarditis
- pneumonia
- arthritis

Your doctor will test you for dry eyes by using what's called the Schirmer's test, where she tucks a small piece of litmus-like paper into your lower eyelid for a few minutes to see how much liquid is emitted from your eyes during the timed test. Testing the salivary glands requires a biopsy—your doctor may or may not order this test, as it's not done as frequently as the less-invasive eye test. Finally, there are blood tests that can be done: Sjögren's usually shows an elevated inflammation level, and often the Ro factor will show up. Most primary Sjögren's patients also show the rheumatoid factor in their blood.

Secondary Sjögren's Syndrome will show all the same symptoms listed above, but everything except the dry eyes, mouth, etc. will actually be associated with whatever rheumatological disease the patient also has.

Sjögren's Syndrome is a little-known and little-understood condition outside of rheumatological circles. When I was first diagnosed with Sjögren's, I had to do a great deal of research about it, as I'd never even heard of it before. I've run into only a few people with Sjögren's since then, but any number of people who have relatives or friends who seem to have been recently diagnosed with it.

Of those people, I hear the same story over and over again: "My friend/relative has to carry a bottle of water with her *everywhere*. Her throat dries out almost instantly." Indeed, that's life with Sjögren's. It's a bother, but it's also serious: If you have Sjögren's Syndrome, you need treatment, medication, and lifestyle changes in order to prevent long-term damage to your body. We'll talk more about what you can do if you have Sjögren's in the next section of this chapter.

Raynaud's Syndrome

Raynaud's will often present itself along with lupus, but sometimes on its own. It's usually carried with patients who have the discoid form of lupus. It is a syndrome where the capillary action doesn't work properly, and so circulation is impeded, especially to the fingers and toes.

Symptoms include:

○ white fingers or toes
○ sometimes red fingers or toes
○ burning in the fingers or toes
○ worse with exposure to cold

Testing for Raynaud's includes a blood test for the rheumatoid factor, though it's not always present in Raynaud's patients. Your doctor will also look at your fingernails under a magnifying glass to see the capillaries. (Mine used the interesting technique of a drop of KY jelly, which then acts to magnify via the dome of the droplet.)

One of the first questions I'm always asked by someone else with Raynaud's is, "What does yours look like?" Everyone's fingers, toes, hands, and feet react differently to having Raynaud's Syndrome. One tech who draws blood for my rheumatologist has Raynaud's. We often compare fingers during the winter, to see whose are more white or more red (mine turn white, while hers turn red). Comparing notes like this is one way of making you feel more normal while having a disease: it's one way of knowing that you're not only not alone, but that others share similar symptoms while developing other symptoms you don't have.

Raynaud's patients who also have lupus are more prone to blood clotting problems than those with lupus alone, as they may carry the

antiphospholipid antibody (or lupus anticoagulant factor). These people will most likely develop deep vein thrombosis (DVT), which is a blood clot that generally forms in the outer limb and moves inward toward the heart and lungs. DVTs are quite dangerous and can kill if not treated in good time. We'll take a more detailed look at DVTs and the lupus anticoagulant factor in Month Six.

Interestingly, one of the early tests for lupus was a syphilis test. Some lupus patients tend to test a false-positive for syphilis. People with Raynaud's Syndrome have a higher chance to test false-positive than people who just have lupus alone.

IN A SENTENCE:

> *Sjögren's Syndrome affects the creation of mucal fluids in the body, while Raynaud's Syndrome affects the body's capillary action, especially to the fingers and toes; both syndromes can be carried alone or with lupus.*

living

Living with Sjögren's and/or Raynaud's Syndrome

MOST PEOPLE will only develop one or the other of these syndromes, either alone or with lupus—or maybe neither of the syndromes. Some of us—me, included—are "lucky" enough to have developed both of them. I refer to what I have as the Family Economy Package: I opted to get them all.

There are some lifestyle adjustments that can and should be made to improve your life with these syndromes, but by and large they won't affect you more than lupus already has.

Life with Sjögren's Syndrome

There are a number of treatments for Sjögren's Syndrome, some of which you can do on your own. Personal and sexual issues will also arise from having this particular syndrome, which you're going to have to work into your changed lifestyle.

TREATING SJÖGREN'S

There are medications on the market for dry eyes and dry mouth, some over the counter. Your doctor will recommend you see an ophthalmologist on a regular basis, because dry eyes, when out of control, can lead to your corneas drying. Dry corneal patches can cause adhesions and even vision changes—you want to follow your ophthalmologist's advice very carefully and dutifully.

There is a medication on the market that your doctor can prescribe called Salagen—this creates moisture for your mouth and eyes, but only for about six hours at a time. You can take the prescription up to four times a day. One caveat, which I've discovered for myself: Don't take it right before bed. Maybe an hour before is best. Why? I tried taking it and then lying down to sleep, and ended up slobbering all over my pillow. It creates quite a bit of moisture when you first take a pill!

There are experimental eye drops out there, being tried by research groups, which are similar to the gel used when you undergo surgery. They're trying to see if the FDA will approve it for day-use in Sjögren's and other dry-eye patients. The outcome of these studies remains to be seen.

KEEPING MOISTURIZED: EYES AND MOUTH

When I was first diagnosed with Sjögren's, I hadn't been given any instructions yet—it was literally the first week we knew I had the syndrome. I woke up one morning with badly burning eyes and so light sensitive that I could barely open them, even though it was a cloudy day. We rushed to the ophthalmologist, scared I was losing my sight. He examined me, and then said I had some dry patches on my cornea that would reverse with adequate moisture, but no adhesions. Then he asked me how often I put drops or gel in my eyes. I told him: never. Turns out that my Sjögren's was particularly active right then, which is how the diagnosis was possible. Luckily, I got good advice from the ophthalmologist about some over-the-counter eye drops and gels that are gentle to the eyes and yet keep them moisturized.

I can't emphasize enough how important it is to keep your eyes moisturized if you have Sjögren's—find some over-the-counter gel that you can use at night, and use it religiously. GenTeal™ makes some great gel that has a gentle preservative that oxygenates (disappears when exposed to air), which I use at night. I also use a nonpreservative saline drop that I can carry in a pocket—they come in capsules that are one-use only and just the right size for one application for dry eyes.

Dry mouth can be just as important to treat: a dry throat can lead to incredibly painful swallowing, burning, and the hazard of adhesions in the mouth and throat. Keep a bottle of water with you at all times; I carry one of those small sports bottles in my purse or in my hand or car. (Note: if you use a reusable bottle, be sure to clean and *purify* it before reusing it. You can get dangerous bacteria buildup if you don't clean sports bottles properly.) Everyone I've met with Sjögren's carries water with them at all times, during all times of year and all types of weather.

Keeping your mouth moisturized helps another cause: your teeth. Because your mouth won't be making as much saliva as usual, plaque can build up more quickly and bacteria can grow that your saliva otherwise naturally staves off. In order to keep your teeth as healthy as possible, you will need to (1) take a medication like Salagen, (2) brush and floss daily after every meal and at bedtime, (3) see your dentist at least yearly for checkups and cleaning. I see my dentist every six months for a cleaning because of my plaque buildup from the Sjögren's. Preventing cavities is crucial for Sjögren's patients.

PERSONAL & SEXUAL ISSUES

Because your bodily fluids are going to be on the low end, you're going to end up with a series of personal issues because of the Sjögren's.

Your breath will be an issue: reduced saliva and dry mouth leads to some nasty breath odors building up. I keep a tin of mints in my purse and in the car at all times; no matter that I've just brushed my teeth, my breath usually needs the extra boost. It's not that you're a bad person to have "dragon breath"; you have a syndrome that causes it, and there's not much you can do about it but try to combat it with brushing after every meal and using breath mints when you need them. Listerine and some other mouth rinses have little gels out on the market that act as breath fresheners, too—give them a try and see what works best for you. Ask a *really* good friend if it's helping; most people will be too polite to tell you that you have bad breath, even your support group. Asking someone to help you out with this can be a great aid—it's hard to smell your own breath effectively.

You may have digestive issues because of the lack of mucal fluids being produced in your small and large intestines. You may need to talk to your doctor about modifying your diet in order to not become either constipated or diarrheal. Gas may become yet another issue for you. Again, your doctor may be able to help, or try over-the-counter gas medicines such as Gas-X.

Finally, if you're a woman, you may have sexual issues because of the lack of fluids in your vagina. Intercourse may become dry and quite painful for you. KY jelly and/or other gels can be used to help lubricate and make up for the lack of fluids. You and your partner need to be carefully aware so you don't literally get hurt by a lack of fluids. Talk to each other about substituting some sort of gel; you may find some that are quite fun!

Life with Raynaud's Syndrome

Raynaud's Syndrome has less personal side effects than Sjögren's, but all the same has effects for which you will need to make lifestyle adjustments.

Because your fingers and toes will get cold very easily, even in warm weather, it's important to keep them warm and/or covered. If you find your toes get cold to the touch even in summer, you may want to wear cotton socks with sandals—it's a very acceptable style in Europe, after all. I tried "toe socks" to see if they kept my toes even warmer and discovered that—at least for me—it had the effect that gloves versus mittens had: my toes were *more* cold if they were separated in the toe socks. Regular socks kept them touching each other, and more warm.

Sometimes your fingers will get white and sometimes bright red. I find that when mine get red, they also become painful to the touch and feel as if they are burning, yet they're cold to the touch. This is the capillary action acting up. There are times you're going to have to simply not use your fingers for typing or other activity when they're really burning badly. At these times, you'll need to educate the people around you as to why your hands are so red and no one can shake your hand, etc. Explaining Raynaud's Syndrome is pretty easy, and most people seem to react positively to a quick explanation.

At times, your fingers will be white and cold and feel as if they're freezing and stiff. At these times, it's important to keep them as warm as possible. I've found that a pair of silk glove warmers (try Winter Silks at http://www.wintersilks.com) act as a thin enough warming glove that I can type, eat, and even sleep with them on and still keep my hands slightly warmer than they were before. When I say slightly, that's because when the Raynaud's is *really* acting up, it feels as if nothing will keep my fingers warm. The important thing is to physically keep them warm rather than rely on how they *feel*—they're going to feel cold no matter what because of the lack of capillary action.

A young man I've met who has Raynaud's wears fingerless gloves to type at his computer. He's still in college and can't get away with adjusting the temperature for his dorm room, but he can adjust to typing with gloves that allow his fingertips to feel the keys. You might want to give them a try if your fingertips aren't too cold without cover of their own.

For my toes, I try to remember to wear my socks—I'm a barefoot kind of person—but I've also been careful to change my lifestyle to accommodate my cold feet. I have one of those foot risers below my desk that not only keeps my legs at the right level for good ergonomics, it also has a blower built into it that can blow warm or hot air onto my feet. Heaven in the winter! At night I wear "bed socks" to keep my feet warm, or they get so cold I can't sleep properly. I've knitted my own, but any loose-fitting sock will do: if you're a knitter, write to me by e-mail and I'll be glad to send you my bed sock pattern (see Appendix).

Because people with Raynaud's are more prone to blood clots (DVTs) than people with just lupus, you will need to make lifestyle changes to make sure you reduce the chance of blood clots forming. When you sit for any length of time, be sure to get up every twenty minutes to half an hour and move around. If you have to sit at a desk, try to elevate your feet on a footstool or footrest. If you're going to sit on a couch to watch a long movie, try to sit with your legs up. Again, try not to sit for any length of time beyond half an hour. If you have to be on a long plane flight, get up often and walk up and down the aisle. I've found that if I explain to the flight attendants that I'm prone to blood clots (and have had them in the past), they are quite accommodating. I've even been able to request the ticket agent book me a bulkhead seat: these are the ones in the very front, up against the bulkhead. I find I can put my feet up on the bulkhead and take a nap quite comfortably there.

Finally, you will want to ask your support group for help with your Raynaud's. They can help pave the way with strangers and new friends via education about your Raynaud's, so people don't ask potentially embarrassing questions in public, such as: "What's wrong with your fingers?!" or "Why are you wearing gloves?" or "Don't you know that socks with sandals look stupid?"

You will need to learn to ignore comments from certain sectors, and lean on your support group when you need encouragement. Raynaud's isn't the worst offender when it comes to lupus syndromes that are physically obvious—perhaps the worst is the lupus mask, which we'll discuss in Month Four. Your friends and family can be of great help with both Raynaud's and Sjögren's Syndromes—don't forget to ask them for support when you think you need it.

IN A SENTENCE:

> In Sjögren's Syndrome, you need to keep up your bodily fluid intake, and for Raynaud's Syndrome you need to keep your fingers and toes warm; but for both syndromes, you need to remember to depend on your support group for help and encouragement.

learning

What is the Lupus Mask?

THE "MASK" that shows up on the faces of some people with lupus, particularly if they have the form of lupus called discoid lupus, is referred to as the **lupus mask**. It is is a skin condition and doesn't affect the health of the patient otherwise.

This masking is clinically referred to as the malar rash, and displays in a butterfly-type pattern over the nose and across the cheeks. For this reason, it's sometimes called the **butterfly rash**, as well.

It can appear red, like a skin rash, or brownish-red, as if the patient had a tan and a rash at the same time. For some people it appears brown or darker, as if they had a raccoon mask rather than the markings of a wolf bite. The illustration on the next page shows the lupus mask as it appears most commonly. Your facial patterns may differ quite a bit, but it's still referred to as a lupus mask.

When lupus was first described as a disease in the thirteenth century, a physician named Rogerius saw the lupus mask on many patients and decided that it looked like a wolf's bite. Hence, the name *lupus,* which comes from the

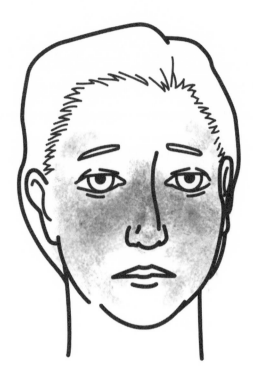

Latin word for *wolf*. Not everyone who has lupus shows the mask, but many patients will show it at least once in their lifetimes, to a greater or lesser degree, especially if they have discoid lupus.

The mask will come and go, just as your lupus flares and goes into remission. Sometimes the mask will appear to be more severe than other times for no reason you can track; it depends on stress levels, your inflammation levels, and the whims of lupus. You may go for years without a mask, then after exposure to sunlight on a bright summer day, you may develop a brownish butterfly pattern over your nose and cheeks, or like a raccoon mask. Then it will disappear again.

Treating the lupus mask

There are few treatments solely for the lupus mask, other than the standard treatments for your lupus, such as NSAIDs, corticosteroids, and immune suppressants. Controlling your flares will help control the mask to a degree. When the mask flares badly and may itch or burn, certain creams can be of help. One of my friends on the Wolfbytes e-mail list has recommended the oatmeal-based creams and cleansers. I was recommended to use Cetaphil to wash with, to prevent disturbing the mask's sensitivity, as it's one of the few completely soap-free cleansers on the market that's made for sensitive skin conditions. It works well for **rosacea**, too, which many lupus patients seem to develop. (Rosacea is a condition where the capillaries in the face are overactive, leading to red skin, burning blushing brought on by heat, alcohol, hot foods, etc., and is often carried by people who have Sjögren's Syndrome.) You can get Cetaphil in just about any drugstore, without a prescription. I've also been lucky in that good, preservative-free, all-natural goat milk soaps work for me in preventing masking irritation: I've been using Zum soaps, from my local natural food market (also at http://www.indigowild.com).

If your mask flares to a great extent and causes irritation, itching, and burning, your doctor will probably put you on a course of corticosteroids or the like, in order to bring down your inflammation levels, which are causing the flareup. Otherwise, treatment is up to you: take care of your skin, keep your stress levels down, and your mask shouldn't bother you too much.

IN A SENTENCE:

> *The lupus mask—also called the malar or butterfly rash—is a skin condition of the face which occurs with discoid lupus.*

living

Life as a Wolf

THE LUPUS mask, as we discussed above, isn't a life-endangering condition of lupus, but socially it's a bear (excuse the bad animal metaphors) to live with. People will look at you, children may point, and you're going to feel like a freak at times. Plus, when it really flares up, the mask can itch and burn.

Let's look at some of the things you can do to help with these issues, particularly the social aspects of living with a "wolf mask."

"What happened to your face?"

The first time I developed the lupus mask, I was at a large professional science fiction/fantasy convention in Minneapolis. I work as a production manager for one of the science fiction publishers, and I was there to socialize with other editors, writers, and friends who work in the field. Unbeknownst to me, overnight I developed the masking. I was late to meet with (coincidentally) Teresa Nielsen Hayden for breakfast, and rushed out of my hotel room without washing my face or looking at it in a mirror. Upon seeing me step out of the elevator and approach her, she looked at me across the large marble lobby of the hotel, and exclaimed in a loud voice that carried throughout the room, *"Nancy, what happened to your face?!"*

I was mortified. I knew instantly that I must have a lupus mask showing. I was a freak. Everyone turned to look at me, of course, after hearing her shout.

I'd just been diagnosed with Sjögren's and Raynaud's Syndromes, and knowing that they often carried the discoid lupus characteristics, I explained to her what was going on, and to some of the people standing around us. To this day, I regret not having a great comeback line, such as, "I thought you invited me to a masked ball!" Oh, well. I'll save that line for another time.

Coping with reactions

This brings us around to coping with the lupus mask, socially. A sense of humor is going to be one of your best defenses against unthinking people who comment on your "face." Annette Bristol, of the Wolf-bytes group, had a child walk up to her in a supermarket one day, stare at her, then say loudly, "What's wrong with your face?" The mother didn't even notice her child's behavior. As I recall, Annette told the child she was really a wolf. That did the trick, and the kid ran off.

People are going to be rude at times—there's no way around it. Many say exactly what they're thinking, without a filter, with the excuse that it's free speech. Free or not, it's rude to comment on somebody's rash or the discoloration on their face. Making a joke back can often break the tension these rude comments engender.

The other defense is education, of course. You don't need to go into detail, but simply say that you have lupus, and lupus means "wolf"—you have a wolf mask, because you have lupus. Especially if it's a child, you can then say, "Do you see the wolf mask? Do I look like a wolf?" Make it into a game: see if the person can "see" how the mask resembles the coloration on a wolf's face. This way you've not only educated, but engaged the adult or child into your world of having a wolf's "face."

Makeup

Makeup is another way to cope with the lupus mask. There are a number of cosmetics on the market, even available at the regular drugstore, that can help tone down redness and the browning from the rash. I've found that the green cosmetics help me less than the yellow ones, but I tend toward more red than brown in my masking. I use a light hand to apply a yellow-colored foundation/concealer from Lorac (Lorac Oil Free Neutralizer), which also calms my skin, then on top of that their oil-free makeup foundation in my normal color—I got this through a Sephora store (also, http://www.sephora.com). If you go to a large cosmetics counter in a department store, ask if their brand has anything for people with rosacea for coverage of the red (since rosacea is far more common than lupus masking). Many companies have colored concealer shades, including Clinique, Awake (Stardom Face Corrector Palette—in white, blue, brown, and yellow), and Benefit (Doctor Feelgood). Look for foundation/primer and makeup concealers, and see if there are any "correcting colors" available in the brand you like to use.

Don't be afraid to do this if you are a man: men wear cosmetics more and more, nowadays, and if you have a rash to cover, it's not at all unusual for a man to ask about coverage foundation. As far as color goes, you're going to have to play with them and find the best coverage for yourself. If you're lucky enough to have a good cosmetologist at your local department store, or you live near a large cosmetics store such as Sephora, ask for help; the men and women who handle cosmetics for a living are very good at what they do, and they'll find something that will help cover the mask without making you look "made up."

Caveat: Some cosmetics may irritate your lupus mask/rash. You should always try just a dab on your rash area first, wait at least five minutes, and see if there is any reaction. If there is, wash it off immediately with an irritant-free soap or cleanser. Strangely enough, the more purely natural the cosmetic, the harsher it can be on easily irritated skin. Many people with rosacea, for instance, can't stand to use makeup from companies such as Aveda, which produces all-natural cosmetics and skin care items.

Be the wolf

If you have discoid lupus and develop the lupus mask, roll with it. Between maintaining a sense of humor about it, covering the rash with makeup as needed, and educating those around you, your mask won't necessarily be the disaster you anticipated. Sure, there are going to be times you feel like wearing a paper bag over your head, or just plain staying in the house with the drapes drawn. Try to jolt yourself out of doing that, however. You can't live in your house forever; eventually you're going to run out of toilet paper, if nothing else. There are people out in the world, possibly even in your neighborhood, with far more obvious facial scars, limps, and even people in wheelchairs with missing limbs. You only have a rash—an annoying rash, certainly, but just a rash.

Living with a lupus mask isn't as bad as it could be: it's not a condition that threatens your life, as other conditions with lupus can certainly do, and it's not usually a condition that stays forever. It will come and go, and you'll learn all sorts of coping mechanisms to deal with it. Have fun: be the wolf.

IN A SENTENCE:

> *Living with the lupus mask can be coped with through makeup, a sense of humor, and educating those around you.*

MONTH **5**

learning

The Pulmonary System and Systemic Lupus

YOUR BODY'S pulmonary system includes your lungs and the tissue surrounding them: the pleural lining. Because your lungs and **pleural lining** are connective tissues, they can be affected by lupus. Typical illnesses that strike lupus patients who have vulnerable pulmonary systems are various forms of **pneumonia**, pleurisy, and **pleuritis** or pleural effusion.

What is pleurisy?

My pulmonary system seems particularly susceptible to lupus conditions. When I first came down with pleurisy, there were several friends—also book production editors— staying with me. I had gone to the doctor complaining of splitting rib pains. He listened, then declared I had pleurisy. "What?!" I said, confused. In my mind, it was a "Victorian disease." The doctor started to spell "p-l-e—" "No, no," I interrupted. "I know how to spell it. I just don't know what it is." Typical copyeditor in me. When I returned home to tell my friends what the doctor told me, both of them piped up, spelling the name of the condition, "p-l-e-u..." but then asked what it *was*. I guess copyeditors are all of a tribe. We can spell just about anything, but we often have to look up definitions.

Pleurisy is an inflammation of the pleural lining around the lungs. It's a large piece of connective tissue—except for the gastrointestinal tract, it is one of the largest connective tissues in the human body. Calling it a lining is a bit of a misnomer. It does indeed surround the lungs and acts as a lining, but it also acts as a sac around the lungs. This means it can fill with liquid, if the inflammation levels in the body rise high enough. When this happens, it's called pleuritis, or a pleural effusion.

Symptoms of pleurisy include:

- sharp pain in the ribs
- chest pain when taking a deep breath
- shortness of breath
- feeling as if you have a broken rib
- your doctor can hear a "pleural rub" on listening to your chest wall with a stethoscope

In fact, "I feel like I've got a broken rib" is the number one sign of pleurisy, unless, of course, you really do have a broken rib. (I once *had* a broken rib, but because I was always in the ER with pleurisy symptoms, the doctors didn't treat the broken rib until after the second X-ray showing it came back. Apologies came from all sectors.)

Pleurisy often comes during cold weather, though you can get a pleural inflammation at any time of the year. During cold weather, pleurisy is usually more acute, as breathing in cold air aggravates the pain you already have from taking in deep breaths.

Treatments for pleurisy are simple: keep warm (for comfort and pain reduction) in the chest area, and take anti-inflammatories (NSAIDs). If you are already on the maximum dose of NSAIDs, and your pleurisy is acute enough, your physician may put you on a short course of corticosteroids, such as a "Medrol pack": a course of 10 days (or more) of Medrol, dosed out in a package to take you up to a maximum dose, then back down again to take you off of it.

Pleurisy isn't life-threatening, but it can be very painful. Most people with pleurisy can kick it in anything from a few days to a few weeks, but sometimes lupus patients report pleurisy hanging on all winter long. Curling up with a warm hot pack—the microwavable bean bags are great—and a comforter is sometimes the best thing you can do when a pleural attack hits.

What is pleuritis?

Pleurisy's bigger brother is pleuritis, or a pleural effusion. When the inflammation grows beyond simply inflaming the pleural lining, liquid can form in the lining sac around the lungs. When this happens, it's called an effusion.

Your doctor can hear the liquid in the pleural lining by listening to your chest wall with a stethoscope. This is a distinct sound from a pneumonial crackle, which is when you have liquid in the lungs themselves. The same symptoms listed above for pleurisy also occur in pleuritis, but can be more painful. In addition, you may feel it's difficult to breathe on one or both sides of your chest, as if you have pneumonia. Unlike pneumonia, however, it won't hurt more if you bend over as versus standing upright—the liquid won't *swoosh*.

The "rub" of pleuritis and its other symptoms will clue your doctor in to treat you with either NSAIDs, as for pleurisy, or more likely with a course of corticosteroids. A pleural effusion, especially if it spreads to both lungs, isn't necessarily life-threatening, but it's more serious than simple pleurisy. More seriously, if untreated the liquid inflammation could spread to your heart, causing **pericarditis** or even a **pericardial effusion**—not something you want to have (see sidebar, next page).

Pleural effusions respond well to treatment and usually subside within a week or two. You will have broken rib-like pain for some time, but your life isn't necessarily in any danger. More than anything else, like pleurisy, pleuritis is just a "real pain"—in this case, in the chest.

YOUR CARDIAC SYSTEM can also be affected by lupus. In the case of your heart, you can develop inflammation in the sac surrounding your heart: the pericardial lining. When it's a simple inflammation, it's called **pericarditis.** When that inflammation turns into liquid filling the sac, it's called a **pericardial effusion**. Both of these conditions are serious and merit attention from a physician immediately, especially if it's an effusion. Symptoms include:

○ chest pain

○ heart attack symptoms, but no sign of a heart attack upon examination

○ lightheadedness when walking, combined with chest pain

○ a history of pleurisy or pleural effusions combined with the above symptoms

Your doctor will put you on a course of corticosteroids after an examination and diagnosis. You will probably undergo a heart ultrasound, which is noninvasive and a simple procedure they'll do in a hospital or clinic setting. If you have an effusion that's particularly serious, affecting the heart itself, your doctor may admit you to the hospital, and they may perform a procedure to drain some of the liquid from the sac surrounding the heart.

What is pneumonia?

A simple definition of pneumonia is liquid in the lungs—one or both. This can be any kind of liquid, but it's usually a clear liquid produced by the body in response to inflammation. Sometimes the lungs will tear a bit inside from heavy coughing from pneumonia, and you will then have blood in the lungs as well—this is hemorrhagic pneumonia. I don't recommend it for fun: coughing up blood is rather startling when it happens, as I found out a few years ago.

Pneumonia can be viral, but it also can be bacterial. When it's viral, you can catch it from another person or even certain types of animals. Bacterial pneumonia is picked up from bacteria in the air: I got bacterial pneumonia once from breathing in the air of a stable that housed a horse that—unbeknownst to us—was suffering from a bacterial pneumonia. Unfortunately, there's nothing you can do to avoid getting

> **BECAUSE LUPUS** patients have a tendency to catch pneumonia easily, you may want to talk to your doctor about an annual PNEUMOCOCCAL INJECTION, to guard against viral pneumonia, especially the winter varieties. These shots are available to the elderly and those with compromised immune systems (such as you).

bacterial pneumonia: it's the luck of the draw. It's easier to stay away from someone with viral pneumonia; at least you know they have it and you can avoid contact while they're contagious.

Pneumonia can be treated by either antibiotics (bacterial), or rest and anti-inflammatories (viral). Both, in fact, require rest. "Walking pneumonia" doesn't mean you get up and walk around with it—it simply means you have a pneumonia that you were walking around with, unawares, until your doctor diagnosed it. Pay attention to proper care during your pneumonia episode and follow your doctor's directions carefully. I ended up with irrevocably torn pleural lining and a partially folded lung after I didn't get proper care during that bacterial pneumonia episode I spoke of above. If your doctor sends you to a pulmonologist (lung doctor) for followup, do everything the specialist says, especially if you're given breathing exercises and the like. It will be important for you to build up your lungs again so they won't be susceptible in the future.

IN A SENTENCE:

> *The pulmonary system (lungs and surrounding tissues) are often affected in lupus patients, leading to the conditions known as pleurisy, pleuritis, and pneumonia.*

living

Pulmonary System Complications in Lupus Patients

LIVING WITH lupus means living with pain. Unfortunately, both pleurisy and pleuritis are quite painful, though not usually harmful conditions. Because the pleural lining around the lungs is such a huge piece of connective tissue, it's often affected by lupus inflammation when your disease flares up. Some people more than others seem prone to getting pleurisy, but no one knows exactly why. Different parts of the body become more vulnerable to lupus flares than others. You'll learn over time what your "soft spots" are. If they're your pulmonary system, then it's a given you'll be down with either pleurisy or pleuritis at one time or another.

When do I call the doctor?

Knowing when to call a professional is a frequent question among lupus patients. In the case of pleurisy, it's often a pretty easy condition to figure out you have. Do you feel as if you have a broken rib, but you haven't done anything to break a rib lately? Does it hurt to breathe deeply? Then you probably have pleurisy. Call your doctor.

Pleurisy isn't going to kill you, but untreated it can lead to a pleural effusion (pleuritis) or even cardiac complications, such as pericarditis. You don't want the inflammation to get out of hand. The first few times you have pleurisy, your doctor will definitely want to see you, so go ahead and call for an appointment. Remember to tell them your symptoms when calling in—they'll probably know immediately that it's pleurisy, but having an examination is important for a lupus patient, just in case it's something more serious.

If you become a frequent flier with pleurisy, it's possible your doctor will let you take up the reins to some extent, if you have that sort of casual relationship with your physician. When I know I have pleurisy, I call my doctor, and she tells me to up my dose of NSAIDs a bit and stay warm and quiet for a few days. If it gets bad, I call for an appointment, especially if I start to have symptoms of either an effusion or pneumonia. She then examines me, and sometimes puts me on a course of Medrol to take the inflammation down before it can become dangerous.

Your doctor may want you to see her every time you have pleurisy symptoms—it all depends on your doctor's methods of practice. Neither way is right or wrong; it all depends on your doctor, and how you and she work together to control your lupus conditions.

But it hurts!

Pleurisy, pleuritis, and pneumonia *hurt*. There's no way around that. Tell your doctor if your pleurisy pain is unmanageable with Tylenol or other pain relievers (NOTE: See sidebar in Week Two: Be careful not to double-dose your NSAIDs!). There are non-narcotic pain relievers available that your doctor may be able to prescribe to get you through the worst of the pain.

Don't forget to keep warm. Warmth will also help with pain relief from pleurisy. I have two of those bean-bag-type pillows you can heat in a microwave. They're actually filled with dried husks that retain heat. You can buy them in stores like Target, or health food stores: you might want to get one that has lavender or another soothing herb inside with the husks, or you might want one that's "unflavored." I have two: one for my ribs and one for my collarbone, since I seem to get aches echoing up there even when the pleurisy is lower in the rib cage. The cats, attracted to the heat, always help me stay warm, of course. A few days on the couch, a couple of hours a day, snuggling with hot packs and a gaggle of cats, and I'm usually feeling much better.

Coughing with pleural pain is the worst—if you have a cough when you have pleurisy or pleuritis, ask your doctor for a cough suppressant. Otherwise, the pain can make you feel as if your ribs are trying to escape from your own chest, á la *Alien*.

How can I prevent pulmonary conditions?

The best prevention against pleurisy, pleuritis, and pneumonia is— for a lupus patient—reduction in stress, and therefore reduction in inflammatory levels. The less likely a flare of lupus, the less likely you'll get pulmonary conditions such as we've discussed. Taking your lupus medications as prescribed by your doctor, reducing stress (visible and invisible) in your life, and using your support group are always your best preventative measures when dealing with this disease and any of its related conditions.

Particularly for pleurisy and its siblings, staying warm in winter and trying to avoid breathing overly cold air seem to help some people in staving off these illnesses. If you have asthma, caring for it and taking your medications daily will be equally important in keeping pleurisy and pleuritis at bay, since the entire pulmonary system interacts. Inflammation in one area can lead to inflammation in another.

It all goes back to what we discussed in Day Four: reduce stress, reduce stress, reduce stress.

IN A SENTENCE:

> *Pleurisy, pleuritis, and pneumonia are painful but not necessarily life-threatening illnesses that can be prevented in lupus patients with proper medications and stress reduction in lifestyle.*

The Lupus Anticoagulant Factor

MANY PEOPLE with lupus, particularly those with systemic lupus, display a blood factor called the lupus anticoagulant factor. This is also referred to as the antiphospholipid antibody. What this means is that lupus patients with the anticoagulant factor tend to have problems with narrowing of the blood vessels and/or blood clots.

If you have this factor, you need to be aware of side effects from it and make some lifestyle as well as medical changes in order to prevent some possibly life-threatening conditions.

What is the lupus anticoagulant?

The lupus anticoagulant is actually an antibody that works as an **autoantibody**: it works *against* the body instead of in favor of it. The lupus anticoagulant is only one of two antibodies found commonly in lupus patients. The other is the **anticardiolipin antibody**. Both of these antibodies are classified as antiphospholipid antibodies. These antibodies can be found in people who don't have lupus, but no one knows why or how some people have one but not the other, or why some people with lupus don't have them at all.

Remember how I mentioned that a **false-positive syphilis test** was also used as a blood test for lupus? That's another antibody that's an antiphospholipid antibody found in lupus patients.

Having antiphospholipid antibodies in your blood means that you're going to be prone to blood clots and other conditions from narrowing of the blood vessels. Your doctor is going to watch out for the following:

- deep vein thrombosis (DVT), or blood clot
- stroke
- heart attack
- poor or slow healing of wounds
- gangrene

If you have these antibodies, you may not get any of those conditions, but you need to be aware of the danger of them, just in case your lupus flares or a situation occurs in which you are put in danger of developing one of those conditions.

How do I know I have these antibodies?

Your doctor will do a series of blood tests to see if you have these antibodies in your bloodstream. One test measures how long it takes for your blood to clot (an activated partial thromboplastin time, or a PTT). Your doctor may also test for the anticardiolipin antibody (IgG, IgM, IgA).

The problem with these tests is that the antibodies will come and go in your system, disappearing for a period of time and then reappearing again for no reason anyone understands. Your doctor should retest you at periodic intervals to see if you test positive for these antibodies if you are showing signs of a tendency toward clotting easily, anemia, or have a history of miscarriages.

What is a Deep Vein Thrombosis (DVT)?

A **thrombolus** (blood clot) that appears in a deep vein in the body, usually the leg, is called a Deep Vein Thrombosis or DVT. This is a blood clot caused by the **hemostasis**—coagulation of blood—being higher or more dense in certain people with lupus, because of the antibodies we discussed above.

If a thrombolus breaks off and travels up the vein, it becomes an **embolus**. This can be a very dangerous condition, as it could travel to the lung and cause what's called pulmonary embolism—this can kill you quite quickly. Treatment for a thrombolus is needed immediately.

Signs of a DVT include:

○ pain in the back of the knee
○ pain in the inside of the elbow
○ pain radiating up the inside of the leg toward the groin
○ sudden swelling of a foot
○ a hot line that runs up the inside of the leg toward the groin (hot to the touch)
○ sudden pain in the lung and inability to breathe
○ symptoms of a stroke

    ○ loss of motor control on one side of the body
    ○ inability to speak
    ○ loss of consciousness combined with the above

If you show these symptoms and have lupus (especially if you already know you have the lupus anticoagulant factor or other antiphospholipid antibodies), CALL 911 and get to a hospital immediately.

DVTs can also affect pregnancy, as a blood clot can lodge in the placenta and cause miscarriages. Often these miscarriages go undiagnosed for a long time, until tests for the antiphospholipid antibodies are run on the patient.

Other blood conditions in lupus patients

Remember that blood works as a connective tissue, which means your blood is affected by your lupus. One such condition is DVTs, as we discussed above. Others include **anemia**, and **leukopenia** and **neutropenia**.

Anemia

Anemia is when you have too little hemoglobin, or red cells, in your blood. You will probably feel very tired, as red blood cells are what carry oxygen to the rest of your body. Most lupus patients develop some anemia at one time or another due to either inflammation levels (a flare of the lupus) or from medications being taken. It can be something as simple as not enough iron in your diet or because you have some gastrointestinal bleeding due to the NSAIDs you take (one of their bad side effects is to cause stomach or intestinal bleeding).

Your doctor will test your blood for red blood cell count and let you know what sort of treatment she wants to approach. Most times it will be trying to reduce inflammation, perhaps with a course of corticosteroids. Other times, she may want to put you on iron supplements. Depending on the severity of your anemia, your physician may have other medications she may want to put you on, including drugs to stimulate your bone marrow to make more red blood cells.

Leukopenia and neutropenia

Both of these conditions can occur when your white blood cells are reduced. Technically, leukopenia happens when your white blood cells are lowered. Neutropenia happens when your neutrophils (or granulocytes) are reduced—these are a type of white blood cell subclass.

Usually your white blood cell count won't go so far down that you're put at risk for increased infections, but sometimes these conditions will flare up. In those cases, your physician will monitor the medications you are taking and perhaps take you off certain ones that can cause the lowering of white blood cells. One such drug is the class of immuno-suppressants. This is why you will have frequent (every six- to eight-weeks) blood tests while you're on those meds.

IN A SENTENCE:

> *Some lupus patients can get blood clots more easily than others because of antibodies in their blood; some also may tend toward low red or white cell blood counts—all are treatable.*

living

Preventing and Living with DVTs

IF YOU are a lupus person who tends toward DVTs or other blood anomalies, you should have your antibodies checked by your physician, as described in the Learning section, above. If you carry the antiphospholipid antibodies, you may need to make adjustments to your lifestyle in order to prevent blood clots from forming.

Life of a DVT: during and after a blood clot

Imagine you have displayed the symptoms of a DVT as described on page 161 in the Learning section of this chapter. You have been taken to a hospital. What now?

A comprehensive medical history will probably be taken, along with blood draws. You will be taken to the radiology department and an ultrasound will be done on your leg (or wherever the DVT seems to be), looking for the clot. When I had a DVT a few years ago, I had had pain in the back of my knee for weeks before my foot suddenly swelled up: we knew what it was immediately. At the hospital, they had to bring in a technician to do the ultrasound—we live in the country, and it was after normal business hours, so she was home at a barbeque! I was nervous that this was all for nothing and that poor woman was dragged away from her family for a ghost pain, but during the ultrasound—there it was! She showed me the DVT on the screen: it was absolutely clear. You could see the blood rushing around a big clot in the middle of the vein. No doubt about it: I had a DVT. Actually, it was fascinating to see the clot on the ultrasound monitor.

You will be checked into the hospital for a minimum of an overnight stay while they start you on blood-thinning medicine. At this stage, it's going to be very important for you to stay *still*. Because mine was in my thigh, it was easy for me to lie down with my leg raised up on about four pillows: it hurt so very much to have it lower, there was no way in the world I was going to get out of bed, even for the bathroom (and I despise bedpans). Besides, with the pain medication they will probably give you, you'll sleep a lot that first day.

The typical blood-thinning medicine given right away is Heparin. This is administered in the hospital in IV (intravenous) format. This medication will not only thin the blood, but help the blood clot form a sort of shell around it, so there is less chance of it breaking off and forming an embolus, which can be very dangerous and life-threatening. If an embolus travels to your brain or lung, you could die very quickly.

In order for you to receive enough Heparin, you will either have to stay in the hospital for a number of days, or you will be given an injectible form of Heparin which is molecularly heavier than the IV form. It needs refrigeration, but can be taken home from the pharmacy and injected into the skin of the stomach in what's called a **subcutaneous** injection (literally, *under the skin*). The needles you'll be given are very sharp and very thin—they're the same needles used for diabetics to inject insulin.

Don't be afraid to inject yourself. Honestly, once you do it, you'll find there's nothing to it. I was stymied by the needles when I was in the hospital, but I was given an ultimatum: I could either learn to inject myself, or I could stay in the hospital for a week. Faced with that choice, I grabbed the needle from the nurse, gritted my teeth, and injected myself. No pain. Nothing to it. A quick jab and you're done. (Note: One trick your nurse may or may not teach you is to gently rub the area where you injected the Heparin. This helps dissipate the liquid. If it stays in one spot, you tend to get little bruises and it can be sore to the touch there for a few days.)

After the course of Heparin is done, you will start on an oral dose of Coumadin, which is a blood thinner taken as a pill. You'll be taking Coumadin for up to six months after a DVT. During that time, you will have frequent blood tests at your doctor's office or clinic to check your clotting levels; the trick is to keep your blood thinner than normal, but not so thin that you'll start to bleed too easily. During the time you're on Coumadin, you won't be allowed to give blood, have surgery (unless it's for a life-threatening situation), and you'll be encouraged to stay away from situations where you could easily cut yourself and bleed. There are certain foods you won't be able to eat while on Coumadin, too—foods and drinks that could either thin or thicken your blood, changing the clotting factors the Coumadin is supposed to balance. Carefully follow your doctor's instructions on what not to eat or do during these months.

Life after a DVT—preventing another one

You may have to change your lifestyle after having a DVT. If you sit for a living (like I do), or you travel on planes a lot, you will need to be careful about elevating your legs whenever possible and getting up to walk around every twenty minutes to half an hour. You need to lose weight, if you're heavy. Extra weight puts more strain on your legs, which means your vascular system has to work extra hard when you move around, and even when you're still. You need to make sure that if you're sick in bed with a lupus flare you don't curl up for too long: elevate your legs with pillows and change positions often.

You may develop pain where the DVT used to be, radiating up the vein that was affected. This is called **Postphlebitic Syndrome**, or

phlebitis. The veins have little gates which regulate blood flow. Sometimes, after a DVT, the gates get confused and "backwash" can happen. This causes pain. In my case, it feels just like the DVT did—same pain, same place—but the pain is much less than the DVT was, and there is no swelling or heat involved. Your physician can refer you to a specialist who can use a hand-powered type of ultrasound in his or her office to check the blood flow in your affected vein.

Unfortunately, nothing can really be done for phlebitis, other than to be careful about elevating your legs, getting up from a seated position often, and wearing special hose/socks that squeeze the calves so the blood flow goes in the right direction. These special stockings are not exactly stylish, but if they'll prevent pain—and perhaps another DVT—and your doctor wants you to wear them, pay attention to your physician's instructions! As we've discussed, a DVT can be a life-threatening condition and is not something to ignore.

Mary, who was my customer service rep at my local bank for many years, had reoccurring DVTs. She was advised to stop her job, which had her sitting in a chair for a living—but she continued working at the bank, sitting for hour after hour. After her third DVT, the blood clot broke off and travelled to her brain. Mary is still alive, but is no longer able to hold down a job, hold a conversation, or even hold her husband's hand. Mary is no longer Mary.

All this is to say, if you have a DVT, *take it seriously.* Do all you can to prevent a reoccurrence, and if it does reoccur, talk to your doctor about what can be done to prevent more. Take all the medications your doctor prescribes for that condition, and (at the risk of repeating myself) *take it very seriously.* I don't want to hear more stories like Mary's in my lifetime—I've had enough friends die of various conditions over the years. If serious illnesses can be prevented, I say go for it.

Support

Overall, you're going to need support. No, not the support hose we talked about above (though you should look into those)! I'm talking about your support group: your friends, family, and outside support for your lupus conditions.

You're going to have times when getting up and around is going to be painful. During a DVT it's incredibly painful and you really can't move at all. I was flat on the couch and in bed for weeks, depending on my husband to bring me everything and help me move, even to the bathroom (I hopped—painfully). I have had bad pain in my life before—I broke my back at one time—but this is a level of pain I hope to never have again. It was a 10 out of 10. Your support group is going to be absolutely necessary if you have a DVT. You really can't take care of yourself during the first few weeks if you've been sent home with injectable Heparin.

When you have recovered, you're still going to need that support of friends and family. Your life is going to be a bit different from now on. If you have phlebitis, during those episodes you will need to have someone help you keep your legs elevated. You may need to take some time to stay still (but don't forget to change positions often!). You will need help with changing your lifestyle, remembering to get up and move around every twenty minutes or so, remembering to ask for special seats on an airplane. Don't be afraid to lean on your support (figuratively or literally) for help with a DVT, both during and after. That's what they're there for, after all.

IN A SENTENCE:

> *DVTs are painful, life-threatening blood clots, but they can be treated and future ones prevented—don't be afraid to ask your support group for help when you have one.*

HALF-YEAR MILESTONE

Now that you're halfway through your first year with lupus, you feel as if you have more control over your life and can rely on your support network for aid.

You have also learned:

O ABOUT SJÖGREN'S AND RAYNAUD'S SYNDROMES.

O ABOUT THE LUPUS MASK (MALAR RASH).

O ABOUT YOUR PULMONARY SYSTEM AND LUPUS.

O ABOUT THE RISK OF BLOOD CLOTS.

Digestive Problems with Systemic Lupus

THE LARGEST contiguous piece of connective tissue in the body is the gastrointestinal system. Because lupus is a disease that causes inflammation in the connective tissues, most lupus patients end up with some sort of irritation or condition of one of the gastrointestinal sections at some point in their lives.

We're going to have a look at what you can do to avoid problems with your gastrointestinal system, help it if there is existing inflammation, changes you can make to your lifestyle, and support systems that can aid you in all of this.

Your gastrointestinal system consists of everything from your throat down to your anus, and everything in between: esophagus, stomach, small intestines, colon, descending colon, and anus. Now you can understand why it's the largest system in your body!

• • •

Diet: what can I eat?

Certain foods and certain ways of eating can irritate your stomach and digestive system more than others. Some people are going to be more sensitive to "hot" (spicy) foods than others. Taking good care of your gastrointestinal system in preparedness for problems is a good idea: a diet high in fiber, high in leafy green vegetables and fruits, and low in fat and harder-to-digest red meats is ideal.

In general, remember that you're probably already taking medicines that make a big (negative) impact on your stomach and digestion: NSAIDs are notorious for causing stomach and intestinal bleeding, sometimes without warning; even the ones that are buffered or time-released can eventually cause problems, if taken long enough and at a high enough dose. Ulcers can form from the irritation NSAIDs cause—your doctor will ask you to keep an eye on any stomach pains that may develop. If they do, you'll have tests done to determine if you've developed an ulcer and changes to your medications may take place.

If you have developed stomach irritation, you'll be asked to stay on an "ulcer" diet: no spicy foods, no tomatoes or other acidic vegetables and fruit (such as oranges and grapefruit), well-cooked foods, and go easy on milk.

Milk is a controversial subject among some people. For some reason, many people with autoimmune and/or rheumatological diseases are also lactose intolerant. In other words, anything with lactose in it—milk, cream, cheese, ice cream—will cause gastrointestinal upset, usually high amounts of gas combined with diarrhea or constipation. I went through several years of hell with gastrointestinal upsets so bad that I ended up in the emergency room on more than one occasion from such high levels of pain I couldn't bear it. Finally, one doctor—on seeing a barium scan showing *huge* pockets of gas throughout my abdomen—suggested I try a lactose-free diet to see if that was the culprit. Sure enough, he was right. Many others seem to find relief from removing as much lactose from their diet as possible. One trick I found out is that if you *must* have cheese, choose the hardest of the cheeses. Apparently, the harder the cheese, the less lactose is in the product. This means Parmesan and romano have little lactose, compared to spreadable brie. Hard cheddar is about middling in lactose. Lactaid™, which is the enzyme you're lacking to help break down lactose in your digestion, can help if you must have some ice cream or milk once in a while, but it doesn't seem to help much for some people. Your doctor can perform a lactose intolerance test, but it's not only long and expensive, it's just plain easier to eliminate the enzymes from your diet and see how it goes. If you get better, then lactose was most likely your culprit.

If you have been diagnosed with Irritable Bowel Syndrome (IBS), there is a great deal of information on diets available. Many people with fibromyalgia seem to have IBS as well, and some lupus patients, too. I highly recommend another book in this series, *The First Year—IBS,* for information on the syndrome, diet plans, and recipes. Heather Van Vorous, the author, also has recipes on her corresponding Web site: www.eatingforibs.com. The government also has a great Web site with recommended dietary information on IBS at: www.4woman.gov/faq/ibs. htm. It lists foods recommended and not recommended for consumption.

Some lupus patients end up with general inflammation of the bowel and are recommended to follow a low-fiber, or easily digestible, diet. It's surprising how many foods you would assume are easy to digest are actually listed as *not* recommended for this diet: peas, for instance are not recommended, but asparagus is okay. The FDA lists a low-fiber diet on the web at rex.nci.nih.gov/NCI_Pub_Interface/Eating_Hints/ eatdiets.html, which is also used by colon cancer patients and the like. The downside of following an easily digestible diet is that you can't eat many raw vegetables or fruits, so you will miss out on some of the nutritional benefits. Tinned fruit just isn't the same: check with your doctor about fruit that can be eaten occasionally to lend more variety and nutrition to your diet. If you are on a low-fiber diet, you need to be careful about vitamins and minerals you'll miss out on from fibrous foods; again, ask your doctor about what supplemental vitamins and minerals you should be taking to compensate for this lack. Losing weight on a low-fiber diet is difficult, too—daily salads just aren't possible, and neither is fresh fruit and bulky "fill-you-up" foods that are low in calories. Check with your doctor about seeing a nutritionist if you need to lose (or gain) weight and are on a low-fiber diet; many insurance plans will pay for nutritional counseling if it is warranted by medical need.

Exercise

Get yourself moving. Lying down, your digestive system has a hard time working; it's not meant to work when you're supine, but when you're upright. Exercise helps your digestive system work better.

The recommended exercise regime by most doctors nowadays includes at least half an hour daily of cardiac movement (something that gets your pulse elevated) and another half hour of stretching and weighted exercise. (Yes, that's more cardiac exercise than recommended even a year ago—it used to be fifteen minutes a day. Doctors are finding that more is better, which is no big surprise to professional athletes and trainers.)

Joining a gym when you have digestive problems may be difficult for you: some people with chronic digestive distress have to have a bathroom quite nearby, without much notice. Going to a gym may cause some concern in that manner. If you have become overweight because of a low-fiber diet, getting out to a gym is equally problematic; no one likes looking "fat" when all the "beautiful people" are working out at their exercises.

You may need to make compromises. If you have to have a bathroom nearby, try exercising at home or at a gym where you have the locker room close to your workout area(s). If you opt to work out at home, try buying an inexpensive recumbent bicycle or a NordicTrack-type of machine, where you can get cardiac exercise daily. Set it up in front of the TV or in the living room, where you can keep an eye on your kids while you work out. By all means, put it where you will *use* it. Do you know how many people have dusty bicycles in their basements? Who wants to go to a damp basement to work out alone beside the washing machine? Make room, if necessary, in a place where you want to use it and feel comfortable working out every single day. You'll need to make this into a ritual, whether it's in the morning or during an afternoon break—but you need to do it every day.

The same goes for stretching and weight-bearing exercise. Because your digestion is wonky, you will need to keep up your muscle strength and build stamina to get you through the bouts that may have you laid up or in the hospital and on your back. Your local sports supply store will carry hand and ankle weights. It doesn't take an expert to use them, but you should ask for some instruction either at your gym or from a local sports instructor or therapist. Get into a regime of using your weights every day, after your cardiac exercise is done. Don't forget to "cool down" with stretching afterward, so your muscles know they can slow down again, so to speak.

If you don't know of a sports instructor or coach, ask at that sports supply store where you bought your hand weights. Or at the gym: most gyms have instructors who also work freelance as coaches. My coach happens to be a massage therapist who works at a clinic that specializes in sports rehab (http://www.gymratgear.com). Now Marv helps me with my weight training, as well as massage for my fibromyalgia aches.

Social situations: what if I embarrass myself?

Living with chronic digestive problems means a life of compromise, to an extent. And some of that compromise is going to consist of social interaction.

When IBS, inflammation of the bowel, or even an ulcer flares up, you may be unable to attend parties, movies, theater, or a concert the way you're used to. You're going to have to pass up on that dip with carrots at the party; you're going to have to make runs to the restroom during a long movie or play; and you're probably not going to feel like slamming in a mosh pit.

The worst situation is when you suddenly, without warning, *need* a bathroom. You're driving down the street in town—what do you do? I've had to rush from my table at a restaurant that didn't have public bathrooms, explain (hurriedly) the situation to the maître d', and seeing the look of terror in my eyes, the proprietor let me use her private restroom for employees. I ran so fast, I can't remember how I got to the back of that restaurant. Most people are understanding, luckily. You may want to rehearse a simple, concise explanation of what your problem is, so you can explain it in a hurry—when needed—to strangers. (I say, "I have an inflammation of my colon from a chronic disease I have, and I *need to use your restroom NOW,* please. Would that be possible?" And I usually look miserable and terrified. No one's ever said no to me. Yet.)

Talk to your doctor if your "urgency" becomes unmanageable; some people with IBS have to talk about solutions to urgency that entail some simple surgery. Most inflammation of the bowel comes and goes in lupus patients, with flares, and can be handled by compromising your social interactions while you're in the throes of a bad time.

Your support group can be of great help in handling these compromises. They can act as educators to other friends of yours as well as strangers, as necessary. They can also help you by supporting you when you want to be out in public during a flare, but need to take it easy and/or use workarounds in order to attend parties, movies, and the like. There will always be people who don't quite understand why you have to go to the bathroom four times during a two-hour movie; a supportive friend can help explain the situation and lessen the feeling of embarrassment on your part.

It's easy to say, "Don't be embarrassed by your behavior when your digestive problem flares up." You're going to be embarrassed. An "accident" may even occur, when you can't quite make it to the restroom in time. These things happen—you have a condition that, while treatable, is going to be chronic. Just as we discussed using a sense of humor about the lupus mask in month four, you will need to develop a sense of humor about your digestive situation. When I had a particularly vicious bout of constipation, crowned by a colonoscopy, I then developed—unexpectedly and suddenly—raging diarrhea in response to the indignities my colon had suffered that week. I *just* missed getting to the bathroom in time. While I waited inside for my husband to bring me a clean pair of underwear, I called to my friends who stood outside the door, hoping I was going to be okay. I shouted, "See? I always told you guys I was full of shit!" Everyone roared, including me.

Laughing about life's embarrassments is sometimes the best way to get through life with lupus.

IN A SENTENCE:

> *Most lupus patients develop some kind of digestive condition during their lifetimes, which can be helped somewhat with diet, exercise, and a good dose of humor.*

learning

Digestive & Bowel Syndromes Associated With Lupus

MANY PEOPLE with lupus end up having some sort of digestive or bowel disorder due to the way the gastrointestinal system works as a huge connective tissue in the body. It stretches almost literally your entire torso, with your small intestine twisting for yards and yards before turning into the colon. Because lupus is a chronic disease that presents as inflammation of the connective tissues, your gastrointestinal system is an enormous target for your illness.

In this section, we're going to take a look at certain conditions that can affect the gastrointestinal system for the lupus patient, how they are diagnosed, and some treatments for these syndromes.

Irritable Bowel Syndrome (IBS)

IBS is a well-known syndrome where the bowel becomes irritated and dysfunctional due to several factors, not the least of which is inflammation. Many lupus patients end up with a form of IBS—to a greater or lesser extent—during their lifetimes. IBS is often caused by stress, which causes more inflammation in the bowel: does this sound familiar?

Irritable Bowel Syndrome causes constipation, diarrhea, pain, urgency to defecate, and difficulties in digestion. The bowel will sometimes stop peristalsis, the waves of movement in the bowel that break down and move matter through the intestines and colon. When peristalsis stops, nothing gets digested; nothing comes out, and the drains back up, so to speak. The bowel will sometimes become inflamed and cause diarrhea, instead, which means you have little nutritional gain from your food, as it's moving through too quickly for proper absorption through the intestinal walls. Sometimes, instead, the inflammation will cause a great deal of pain in the colon—which has nerve endings inside it—whenever anything passes through; it makes matter going through feel like broken glass. Finally, it can also create an urgency to pass your bowels: almost no warning is given before you will feel that you need to go to the bathroom *immediately.* As we discussed in the Living section, above, this doesn't make for much fun in life.

IBS can be treated with drugs, such as corticosteroids for reduction of inflammation, and motility medications. You will certainly be recommended to a gastroenterologist—a doctor who specializes in the digestive system—if IBS is suspected. A colonoscopy or sigmoidoscopy to see what's going on inside is usually required; your doctor or gastroenterologist will talk to you about how he or she would like to diagnose and track your IBS. Diet is especially important in treating IBS. Again, I highly recommend the books by Heather Van Vorous, *The First Year—IBS* and *Eating for IBS.*

Neuropathy of the colon

If true IBS isn't diagnosed, you may have neuropathy of the colon. In this case, the colon has become inflamed to the point where the nerves are damaged and either no longer function correctly or are hypersensitive. The colon—especially the descending colon, which leads down the left side of your abdomen to your anus—depends on its nerves for proper peristalsis and letting you know when matter hits the end of the descending colon and needs to be eliminated. If these nerves are damaged, you will either have pain and spasms every time there is matter in the colon, or you will have spasms and a sense of urgency, since the descending colon will be unable to properly alert you of the need for elimination. You may have all sensations at the same time: pain, spasms, and urgency. This is why we discussed handling social situations in this month's Living section, above; neuropathy of the colon means making compromises in your social life.

Diagnosis of this condition follows along the same line as that for IBS, which Heather Van Vorous covers fully in her book. In short, a rectal exam is usually followed by a colonoscopy or sigmoidoscopy, in which the doctor examines the inside of the colon using a flexible tube on which is mounted a camera. He may take samples of the colon wall or any suspect areas he sees. If you have neuropathy of the colon, he will see inflammation that can't necessarily be attributed to any other cause; it will be consistently there every time it's examined, and it won't have polyps or other conditions associated with it. Just inflammation and nerve damage that can't be explained otherwise. Motility will be impaired, which will also show on exam.

Treatment includes anti-inflammatories, including buffered NSAIDs, and corticosteroids as necessary during flares. Motility drugs will be used to help make up for the nerve damage. Unfortunately, once this damage is done, it's generally permanent: you will most likely need treatment for the rest of your life. But if you keep your diet to a low-fiber consistency, rest well, keep your stress levels down, and are good to your digestion, you should be able to keep the flares under control—just as you keep your lupus flares controlled.

Your gastroenterologist is your friend

Lastly, I'd like to recommend that if you do develop any gastrointestinal problems, you seek out a good gastroenterologist. If you don't get good results—if he or she doesn't listen to you, recommend stress reduction over heavy medications, and you don't feel as if he is giving you enough time for questions—find another one. You will depend on your gastroenterologist every time you have a bad flare, and you don't want more damage done to your system with a badly controlled or uncontrolled flare of the inflammation.

Talk to others in your support group, asking for recommendations of a good gastroenterologist. Talk to your primary care physician about referrals. Make sure your recommended doctor is not only board certified, but board certified specifically in gastroenterology. Make sure he is up to date on his research. Check and see if he has other patients who have lupus and your particular gastrointestinal syndrome. You want to know that he deals daily with your condition and doesn't concentrate his reading and research on, say, just colon cancer instead.

It all goes back to what we discussed earlier in this book: You are in charge of your medical care. You need to have a good rapport with your physician and feel comfortable with his or her working style. You two are going to be partners in a long-term relationship that's called lupus.

IN A SENTENCE:

> IBS, *neuropathy of the colon, and other gastrointestinal syndromes are linked with lupus because of their inflammatory condition; a good gastroenterologist will help you diagnose and treat these syndromes.*

living

Being Kind to Your Kidneys

KIDNEY DISEASE (**lupus nephritis**) is often linked to lupus, since the kidneys are yet another connective tissue that can be affected by lupus, and many medications taken by lupus patients can adversely affect kidney function.

Let's take a look at how you can help your kidneys to prevent damage to them, and how you can help if you're already suffering from lupus nephritis.

Medications: *making compromises*

Many medications we take for lupus can have an adverse effect on the kidneys. In particular, nonsteroidal anti-inflammatories (NSAIDs) and drugs containing salicylate (aspirin) can be very harsh on the kidneys and cause fluid retention (edema) and some loss of kidney function (such as spilling ketones, or protein, into the urine).

In the cases in which lupus patients develop loss of kidney function due to medications, most of the time the effects can be stopped and even reversed by halting the drug. In these cases, however, what's happened isn't true kidney disease or nephritis. The problem, of course, is that most lupus patients need to be on NSAIDs or aspirin to work as anti-inflammatories: compromises will have to be made. If the kidney function isn't too bad, some doctors will put their patients on short courses of dieuretics to reduce the fluid retention, so they can keep taking their NSAIDs. Others will try to have the patients ramp down on their NSAIDs as much as possible without losing the benefits needed for inflammatory response from the lupus.

Diet: eating right for your kidneys

Another compromise to help fight loss of kidney function due to either nephritis or medication-induced kidney disease is diet. Cutting down on salty foods, watching fat intake, and protein balance are important.

With high-protein, low-carb diets (such as the Atkins Diet) being so popular nowadays, I feel I need to make a couple of comments on this type of diet for the lupus patient. First of all, I'm not a dietician, and I'm not a doctor. But those dietitians and doctors consulted, including your own, will all agree that a high- to all-protein diet for lupus patients is a "bad idea." *Higher* protein, such as the diet proposed by the American Diabetes Association, isn't so bad, but all-protein is iffy for those who run the danger of kidney disease and dysfunction.

High-protein diets work by stuffing the body with so many proteins they begin to spill into the urine as ketones—this state is called **ketosis**. In ketosis, your kidneys have reached their limit in processing protein you've eaten and are now pushing the protein out into your urine in a last-ditch effort to get it out of your body. This stresses the kidneys and, in fact, is the state you are trying to *avoid* as a lupus patient. Ketosis is a stage of *kidney dysfunction* and a stage you can reach if you're in kidney failure due to disease. Creating this situation for yourself is not an ideal way to treat your body.

Balancing your protein and carbohydrate intake, instead, is an ideal for the lupus patient, and can be done with a little good research and/or the aid of a dietitian. As we discussed earlier in this book, your insurance company may even pay for counseling with a dietician if your doctor can show it is necessary medically. If you are in danger of kidney dysfunction, this is definitely a medical necessity, if you and your physician can't come up with a good diet plan between yourselves. The old-fashioned "pyramid" of eating (see www.usda.gov/cnpp/images/ pyamid.gif *or* www.usda.gov/cnpp/pyrabklt.pdf) is a good place to start, as is the slightly modified pyramid that places a bit more protein on the bottom, but doesn't overdo it. Carbs and protein are still balanced in this scenario, with fat still being your least-eaten food group.

Reducing salt is also important. I know, salt *tastes* so good to so many people. But it also places stress on your kidneys, as the kidneys try to filter the salt and eliminate it from your body (think of your kidneys as the oil filters of your body, if you were a Buick). The more salt you eat, the more stress you put on your kidneys. Reducing salt in your diet is reasonably easy nowadays; there are so many low-salt products out on the market. The trick is getting used to the taste of reduced or no salt. I've had little salt in my food for so long now, that I find I can only bear a little bit of it at a time. For instance, regular soy sauce tastes so salty to me, I can't stand to use it with my sushi anymore. It overpowers the taste of anything else!

If you're addicted to cooking with salt, try some of the more flavorful salt substitutes out there, such as Mrs. Dash, when you're broiling meat. Or a little cumin in your chili, or lemon thyme in your green beans. It's amazing how many herbs and spices are available fresh and dried. One trick: Your local health food market will have more flavorful dried herbs than the supermarket, as they don't sit on the shelf for as long, and aren't preserved with stabilizers. You'll want to replace the green herbs at least every six months, but others (like curry powder) will keep for years if kept in a dark, dry pantry.

IN A SENTENCE:

> *Possible modification of your lupus medications and keeping a healthy diet are important to help prevent and treat kidney disease and dysfunction.*

learning

Lupus Nephritis and Other Kidney Dysfunction

KIDNEY DISEASE and kidney problems occur in about one third of all of those with lupus, at some time during their lives. There are various levels of kidney involvement, a couple of different reasons kidney disease can occur, and several ways of diagnosing and treating lupus nephritis.

Diagnosing lupus nephritis

First of all, your doctor will try to determine if you are spilling protein into your urine. He or she may do this long before there are any symptoms showing, such as swelling— or edema—in your legs and feet. You will give a urine sample, and it will be checked for ketones, or protein. If you are spilling protein, then your physician will try to determine whether this is being caused by kidney disease or rather if it may be caused by medications you are on, such as NSAIDs (see Living section, above). If he suspects your medications are causing protein spillage, then he may try cutting back on the drugs to see if the problem corrects itself.

Often, the first sign of kidney dysfunction is edema in the legs and feet, caused by fluid retention. This is actually the second stage of the disease, and is caused by the protein spilling from your kidneys. Sometimes a person will develop edema, a urinalysis (urine test) will be done to check for protein, and only low percentages of protein will show up. If the protein then comes and goes, the nephritis is quite mild, and often little needs to be done other than keep checking periodically to make sure that it doesn't get worse suddenly. If you are in this position, your physician may put you on a course of medication to help with fluid retention, but not much more.

Patients with lupus nephritis are also at a higher risk for developing blood clots (DVTs), such as we discussed in Month Six.

Because the primary symptom of kidney disease is protein spillage into the body's systems, two types of tests can be done to determine the level of nephritis: urinalysis and blood work.

URINALYSIS

Standard urine tests can be performed to see how much protein and/or blood is being spilled into the body's urine from kidneys that are unable to handle their job of filtering waste and fluids. Protein in the urine is called proteinuria, red blood cells in the urine is hematuria, and white blood cells in urine is leukocyturia.

Another method is to collect urine over a period of twenty-four hours to see how well the body is (or is not) filtering protein and fluids. A graph is plotted to see how the body passes protein or blood off into the urine during an entire day.

BLOOD TESTS

There are several tests that can be done to diagnose lupus nephritis by checking for certain telltales in the blood. Some tests can show antibodies that turn up in nephritis patients, and another (the serum complement test) measures certain proteins in the blood that are lower in lupus nephritis patients.

Spilling protein into urine may mean your blood will show a lower protein count, which can also be measured through a simple blood test. Fluid retention (edema) will mean your salt, potassium, and water levels in the blood will also be off normal—these are determined through several blood tests.

OTHER TESTS

An X-ray can be taken of the kidneys, after a contrasting dye is injected into an IV, which will show an outline of the kidneys. A biopsy can also be done (sometimes referred to as a needle biopsy) with a needle inserted into your back and a small portion of kidney is then removed. A sonogram can also be done, where sound waves are sent through the body and an image of the kidneys shows up on the computer screen.

Treatments for lupus nephritis

As we discussed in the Living section, above, diet and exercise are used to help prevent nephritis as well as a supplemental treatment of mild kidney disease. In addition, mild kidney disease and its effects can be treated with diuretics to reduce excess fluids (edema), blood pressure can be reduced through antihypertensive medicines, and anticoagulation drugs such as aspirin or Coumadin can be prescribed for blood clots that occur from kidney disease.

Just as regular severe lupus is often treated by medication that helps control the immune system's over-responsiveness that characterizes lupus, lupus nephritis is also treated in the same manner. Corticosteroids are used in long-term or high-dose courses to help lessen the effects of the kidney disease, though sometimes the side effects can interfere with the patient's overall health—including a higher risk for infection, more fluid retention, and loss of bone mass. Immunosuppressants are also used to block the immune system's response, which is causing kidney damage. In general, corticosteroids are used in earlier nephritis, while a combination of them with immunosuppressants are used with more severe, later-stage kidney disease.

If the kidneys fail to function, dialysis can be done to help the patient: this procedure uses a machine to filter the patient's blood through it, to remove waste that the kidneys would otherwise process themselves. Eventually, those with kidney failure can and should have kidney replacement through a transplantation surgery. Because people with lupus are a higher risk for organ rejection and secondary conditions that could affect the new kidneys, doctors will usually keep a lupus nephritis patient on artificial dialysis until any signs of active lupus are gone, then put them on the list for organ transplantation surgery.

IN A SENTENCE:

> *Lupus nephritis—kidney disease—is a serious form of lupus that can be diagnosed via blood and urine tests; it is treated by medications commonly used by lupus patients, but full kidney failure will require dialysis and eventual organ transplantation.*

Sleep Disorders

MOST PEOPLE who suffer from lupus, as well as those who have overlapping syndromes—particularly fibromyalgia—also suffer from sleep disorders. A sleep disorder is anything that constitutes a disruption in normal sleeping patterns, including too much or too little sleep. Pain is the number one cause of sleep disorders, but there are a number of other culprits that can cause disruption in sleep.

Sleep disorders in lupus patients

Many lupus patients have a hard time sleeping, or feel as if they aren't getting enough sleep. Some feel as if they're getting too much sleep. Others feel as if they're sleeping an adequate amount of time, and yet continue to be fatigued. All of these conditions can be attributed to sleep disorders, if other factors have been discounted.

There are a number of diseases and syndromes that are associated with the mechanisms of sleep, including narcolepsy, sleep apnea, chronic fatigue syndrome, and fibromyalgia. We're going to look specifically at syndromes that seem to overlap with lupus more often than not, rather than examine separate diseases such as narcolepsy or even Kleine-Levin Syndrome (a rare sleep disorder in which the patient sleeps excessively and enters a state of trance when "awake").

FIBROMYALGIA

As we discussed in Day Six, many people with lupus also have fibromyalgia, which is a rheumatoid disease but not an autoimmune disorder, like lupus. Fibromyalgia is marked by pain throughout the body, particularly in the "trigger point" areas, illustrated on page 71.

Fibromyalgia pain is continuous, but seems to be aggravated by its congruent sleep disorder—the fibromyalgia patient can't seem to fully relax all the muscles during sleep cycles because the pain in those muscles keeps them just "awake" enough to constantly tense them, even unconsciously. Most fibromyalgia sufferers aren't even aware that they're not adequately falling into a deep sleep cycle—particularly REM, or rapid eye movement, cycles, which is when we dream—and so often don't report sleep disturbances to their physicians.

The REM cycle is important to restful sleep; without it, we can't get adequate rest no matter how often we sleep or for how long. Studies have been done to artificially suppress the REM cycle of sleep in human subjects. In those studies, the subjects fell into a pattern of severe sleep deprivation behavior very quickly, even though they were "sleeping" normal hours. They became irritable, complained of pain, exhibited reduced ability to suppress emotions, were unable to think clearly, and even developed hallucinations and other psychotic behavior.

The fibromyalgia patient who develops a pattern of reduced REM sleep ends up with more pain, and less REM sleep, which leads to more pain and even less REM sleep, cycling into a pain-sleep disturbance pattern that is difficult to break.

DEPRESSION

Many lupus patients experience clinical depression at some point in their lives. According to the Lupus Foundation of America, 15–60% of people with chronic diseases suffer from depression. Some of the depression is environmental—i.e., it is caused by the fact that the patient has a chronic illness and is therefore depressed about being sick. Some of the depression is clearly not environmental, however, and is most probably organic—i.e., it is caused by chemical changes in the brain, triggering depression. Often it is the serotonin uptake receptors in the brain that either fail to trigger or fail to produce enough serotonin for proper functioning.

Symptoms of depression include (from LFA brochure, "Depression in Lupus" by Howard S. Shapiro, M.D., 1998):

- sadness and gloom
- spells of crying (often without cause)
- insomnia or restless sleep, or sleeping too much
- loss of appetite, or eating too much
- uneasiness or anxiety
- irritability
- feelings of guilt or regret
- lowered self-esteem
- inability to concentrate
- diminished memory and recall
- indecisiveness
- lack of interest in things formerly enjoyed
- fatigue
- headache
- heart palpitations
- diminished sexual interest and/or performance
- body aches and pains
- indigestion
- constipation
- diarrhea

One of the primary symptoms of depression is sleep dysfunction. The patient will either sleep far more than usual, but without receiving a "refreshing" sleep, or will suffer from a form of insomnia—the inability to sleep. Most lupus patients exhibit sleepiness from pain, chronic fatigue, or other conditions, but depression should be examined as a possible cause. Luckily the treatments for fibromyalgia pain and depression are similar: certain antidepressants seem to be very effective. We'll talk more about treatments under the next section: Living.

SLEEP APNEA

Apnea means a suspension of breathing—not breathing for a short period of time. When this happens during sleep, it's called *sleep apnea.* One of the causes of sleep apnea is weight gain; those lupus patients who are on a long-term or high-dose course of corticosteroids often gain quite a bit of weight in a short period of time. The resulting extra tissue in the back of the throat from such weight gain can cause sleep apnea.

During sleep, a person suffering from sleep apnea will have anywhere from a few to several hundred episodes of very short—sometimes only a second or two—periods when breathing is stopped. The person will then gasp, opening the throat again, and start breathing again. Loud snoring and this gasping sound are usually the obvious cues that sleep apnea is occurring. Because these episodes are so short, the person suffering from sleep apnea will come out of deep or REM sleep, almost but not quite waking to consciousness each time the apnea happens. Sometimes the person will actually wake up fully, if he or she gasps enough. Sleep is obviously disturbed by all this behavior; the person with sleep apnea will not get anything close to a restful night's sleep, no matter how long he or she actually sleeps.

Someone with sleep apnea will start to develop signs of sleep deprivation, including daytime fatigue (usually severe fatigue), irritability, difficulty concentrating, and will fall asleep in the middle of sentences. The level of sleep deprivation, plus oxygen being blocked from the brain during the episodes when the person doesn't breathe, means that sleep apnea is actually a very serious condition.

Sleep apnea is a dangerous condition and should not be ignored. Those who have sleep apnea are in danger of brain damage from lack of oxygen, and heart attack. A friend of mine, Bruce, has sleep apnea, and still sloughs off any suggestion that he needs to be seen by a doctor for it. He keeps feeling as if the major problem the apnea causes is the loud snoring, which he says annoys his girlfriends. If he keeps ignoring the apnea, though, he may not have many more girl-friends: he may die from the apnea itself (*Hear that, Bruce?!*).

If you suspect you have sleep apnea, contact your physician as soon as possible. He or she will probably refer you to a clinic or center for sleep study—often these are housed at a local hospital. There they will conduct a study to see how you sleep during a night, measure your heart with an EKG monitor, measure your brain functions with an EEG monitor, and measure your breathing. Depending on how the study goes, recommendations will be made for either surgery or the use of a CPAP machine, which blows measured positive air pressure into your nose and/or mouth during sleep to keep your airways open.

CHRONIC FATIGUE

As we discussed in Day Seven, clinical chronic fatigue—as well as Chronic Fatigue Syndrome, or CFS—often accompanies lupus. The feeling of fatigue can be overwhelming for some lupus patients, lead-ing to a cycle similar to that experienced by those with fibromyalgia: pain leading to sleep dysfunction, leading to more pain, leading to more sleep problems, in a vicious cycle.

Chronic fatigue is distinguished from simple tiredness in that it lasts for a certain period of time without letting up, and it disrupts your nor-mal course of life. The feeling of being tired never goes away, no mat-ter how much sleep you get. Chronic fatigue is diagnosed after all other sleep disorders are dismissed as possibilities, as it can mimic many of the sleep disorders. In a way, chronic fatigue (like fibromyalgia) is diag-nosed by what it is *not* rather than what it *is*: your doctor will try to determine if you have other sleep problems first, then if nothing else fits the bill and you still have overwhelming fatigue lasting for weeks at a time, he or she will probably diagnose chronic fatigue associated with lupus, or Chronic Fatigue Syndrome itself. Since both are treated the same way, there's little difference in the diagnosis in the end.

RESTLESS LEG SYNDROME

No one knows what causes restless leg syndrome, but it seems to affect a number of people with rheumatoid and/or autoimmune illnesses. Restless leg syndrome is when your legs have the need to move and bend, to relieve an overwhelming urge or even pain. It worsens at night. Because it happens in your sleep, you will have interrupted REM and deep sleep, leading to sleep deprivation, very much like that which happens in fibromyalgia pain during sleep. You will waken with the bedcovers disarrayed from your legs moving in your sleep; you may wake up fully in your sleep with a feeling that you must move your legs, or that your legs feel painful and need to be moved to relieve the pain.

Diagnosis of restless leg syndrome consists of eliminating other sleep disorders and sometimes a sleep study at a clinic for observation of the patient during sleep. There are medications—mostly antidepressants—that seem to work to help reduce the urge to twitch and move the legs during sleep.

CHRONIC PAIN

Lastly, chronic pain as a general category needs to be mentioned in conjunction with sleep disorders. People with lupus often live in chronic pain during flares and sometimes even in between flares, depending on the severity of their lupus and how the disease is presenting itself.

If, for instance, you have developed pleurisy (see Month Five), the pain in your ribs and pleural lining will keep you awake at night, disrupting what rest you can try to get. The same goes for many of the conditions and syndromes lupus manifests: pericarditis is painful, a blood clot and its aftermath—postphlebetic syndrome—is quite painful, arthritis can keep you awake, or at least disrupted, during the night. If you develop Bell's Palsy, sleeping can be difficult, as one eye usually can't close anymore—taping it is a solution, but I can tell you from personal experience that it disrupts your sleep anyway.

ACID REFLUX DISEASE

Many lupus patients end up developing stomach conditions from taking NSAIDs for a long period of time. Acid reflux disease is one such

What Is Bell's Palsy?

BELL'S PALSY is an inflammation of the seventh cranial nerve, affecting one side of the face. That side of the face becomes paralyzed, to a greater or lesser degree, depending on the severity of the inflammation. It most often occurs in people between the ages of 30–60, and is more likely to occur in someone who has an inflammatory disease, such as arthritis or lupus.

A person who develops Bell's Palsy will often literally wake up one morning and notice one side of their face sagging when viewed in the mirror, or when smiling or frowning, the mouth doesn't quite move up and down properly. In my case, I noticed over a period of several days that I started dribbling when trying to drink from a coffee cup; my lip would not properly shape to the cup edge.

A neurologist is usually recommended by your primary care physician, to make sure the palsy isn't anything more serious. Bell's Palsy is usually treated with anti-inflammatories or Prednisone (corticosteroid) if the palsy doesn't reverse all by itself. Most times, the palsy will simply go away all by itself within a matter of weeks or months. In my case, it was gone within two weeks without any use of medications.

condition that can show up. This is when the stomach produces more acid, for digestion, than is needed, and the acid refluxes (rises up the esophagus), causing pain and burning—and eventually damage to the esophagus.

Acid reflux is worse at night, because you are lying down. If you have acid reflux disease, you may find that stomach pain will wake you at night, as well as the burning and pain from the reflux. This pain can be excruciating, almost resembling a heart attack.

Acid reflux is nothing to sneeze at: it can erode your esophagus, cause damage to your digestive track, and even cause you to develop asthma from the reflux up your throat. You should talk to your physician if you find yourself with "heartburn" that doesn't go away or consistently becomes worse during the night. Your primary care physician will probably refer you to a gastroenterologist, who can treat you for acid reflux disease with medications that suppress the stomach's ability to produce acid, after he or she diagnoses you.

IN A SENTENCE:

> Sleep disorders can be treated with a combination of medications and lifestyle changes—you can learn to sleep well, no matter the disorder.

living

Coping with Sleep Disorders

LIVING WITH a sleep disorder takes work, both on the part of the patient, and on the doctor's end, as he or she endeavors to make a diagnosis, sometimes with one or more sleep disorders or factors that could cause the disorders overlapping in the lupus patient.

Many of the treatments for sleep disorders are the same, depending on the syndrome. We'll take a look at some treatments for the disorders we discussed in the first part of this chapter, as well as some overall hints that can help most people with sleep dysfunction.

Treatments

If you have fibromyalgia, your physician will probably recommend the same sort of medications for treatment of the sleep disorders these conditions can cause.

The type of NSAIDs (nonsteroidal anti-inflammatories—see Week Two) that are called COX-2 inhibitors seem to provide more pain relief without stomach upset. Remember how we talked about acid reflux disease, above? That's something to be avoided, and not just because it can cause sleep dysfunction. These same COX-2 inhibitors can help with sleep by dulling your pain from fibromyalgia or lupus conditions such as pleurisy.

You may also be prescribed antidepressants: depression and fibromyalgia both need the serotonin elevated in the brain, one to elevate mood and the other to improve sleeping in fibromyalgia. Two different types of antidepressants are usually prescribed:

- tricyclics (amitriptyline—Elavil) (doxepin—Sinequan)
- SSRIs, or selective serotonin reuptake inhibitors (fluoxetine—Prozac) (paroxetine—Paxil) (setraline—Zoloft)

A muscle relaxant that is also an antidepressant is also sometimes prescribed for fibromyalgia: cyclobenzaprine (Flexeril).

Depression is usually treated with the same sort of antidepressants fibromyalgia uses, though sometimes anti-anxiety drugs and others are also used in order to relieve the depression caused by low serotonin levels in the clinically depressed. Depression is also treated with higher doses of antidepressants than are generally used for fibromyalgia patients.

Sleep apnea is treated with surgery that removes excess tissue in the throat. There are two sorts of surgeries that can be done: radical, which removes the tonsils, adenoids, glottis, and excess tissue in the upper palette and throat; and a laser technique, which shaves the excess tissue with precision. The other option, and the one generally tried first, is use of a CPAP machine—a positive air pressure machine with a mask that fits over the nose (and sometimes mouth), blowing air into the throat as you sleep, keeping the tissues open and preventing them from closing over, causing apnea. If a CPAP machine can't be used, or doesn't work, then surgery is often an option.

In lupus, clinical chronic fatigue's symptoms can be alleviated through the use of Plaquenil (an antimalarial drug used to treat arthritis and lupus symptoms), though if the patient can't tolerate Plaquenil—say, he or she developed Plaquenil retinopathy and had to terminate use of the drug or risk eyesight loss—then the use of some of the immuno-suppressants used in lupus can sometimes help with fatigue. Imuran is one such immunosuppressant that seems to help with chronic fatigue symptoms in lupus. Chronic Fatigue Syndrome (CFS), on the other hand, is generally treated with antidepressants in similar doses to those for fibromyalgia.

How can I sleep well?

Everyone agrees that there's nothing as good as a good night's sleep. But how to get such a thing if you have a sleep disorder?

There are a number of tips from different sources on how to improve sleep conditions, many of which you can find on the Internet or from pamphlets your doctor's office has on hand. The Arthritis Foundation has eight tips for sleeping better, from their pamphlet on "Fibromyalgia":

- Make your bedroom as comfortable and as quiet as possible. Invest in a good mattress. Maintain a comfortable room temperature.
- Use your bedroom only for sleeping and for being physically close to your partner.
- Avoid caffeine or alcohol before bedtime.
- Take a warm bath before going to bed.
- Avoid long naps. If a nap is needed to get you through the day, keep it short and schedule it well in advance of your bedtime.
- Read before bedtime, if you like, but avoid suspenseful, action-filled novels or work-related material that can preoccupy your thoughts and cause a poor night's sleep.
- Eat a light snack before bedtime. You should not go to bed hungry, nor should you feel too full.
- Set aside time before bed for relaxation.

I can attest to the last item: I work at home—as do many people with lupus and its related syndromes, in order to accommodate a less stress-ful lifestyle—and often work right up till the time I need to go to bed. I've learned that no matter how "tired" I feel as I finish my work for the day, I need to take about half an hour to unwind and stop my mind from thinking about work. I take a cup of water, my bedtime medicines, a few nuts or snacky food, and sit down to watch a favorite TV show or read a magazine that's unrelated to work. I "just look at the pretty pictures," as I often tell friends. It's my time to *not* think.

The same goes for time when I lie down in bed. I try very hard not to go over the day in my mind or think about the next day's activity. But I'm a workaholic, and I'm a natural thinker—I unwind everything and try to figure out every nuance. It drives my friends crazy. And it could keep me awake, but for a trick a friend taught me years ago. It's an old meditation technique to be used to fall asleep, and it seems to work for me, at least. If you find yourself reviewing the day, make it into a structure process instead. Go through the entire day backward, detail by detail, seeing in your mind's eye exactly where you were, who you were with, what you saw, what you did, what you said. Try to picture it all very carefully and in as much detail as possible, including the words said between you and others. By the time you get to the previous morning's events, you should be either fast asleep or close to it. I usually fall asleep by the afternoon—I don't usually make it as far as the morning. I've also found that that particular meditation also makes for some interesting dreams which help me work out any problems I had during that day. I usually wake up in the morning with a solution in my head.

If you continue to have problems relaxing in bed or before bed, talk to your doctor about learning some meditation techniques. Your insurance company may pay for hypnosis sessions, where you can learn self-hypnosis techniques wherein you can talk yourself into sleeping, or even yoga classes that can teach you both relaxation for mind and body as well as good exercise.

IN A SENTENCE:

> *A number of conditions shared by lupus patients can cause sleep disorders, including fibromyalgia, chronic fatigue, depression, sleep apnea, restless leg syndrome, chronic pain, and acid reflux disease.*

Can I Get Pregnant & Have a Healthy Baby?

TRADITIONALLY, DOCTORS advised against women getting pregnant if they had lupus, but times have changed, and with adequate preparation and medical help, women with lupus can have safe pregnancies with healthy babies.

We'll take a quick look at improving your pregnancy if you have lupus, what precautions you can take, and what compromises you're going to have to make in order to have a good pregnancy.

Most importantly, you will need to *plan your pregnancy* if you have lupus. Compromises and some hard decisions await you.

Improving your pregnancy

The best time to get pregnant is when you are not having a flare. If you can time it so that you know you'll probably have a good window of nine months without a flare, that's ideal. If your lupus isn't as predictable as that (and most aren't), all you can do is try for pregnancy during a flare-free window, then try to stay healthy during your pregnancy by following the usual health tips for lupus patients:

- eat well
- sleep well
- reduce your stress as much as possible
- exercise in moderation but consistently
- take your medications as prescribed
- don't drink alcohol
- don't smoke
- don't take recreational drugs

You're going to have flare-like symptoms during your pregnancy, such as edema (fluid retention) in your legs and feet, the feeling of muscle aches and pains, and fatigue, but these are all symptoms that also go along with a normal pregnancy. It's going to be difficult to tell the difference, but your physician can help you sort out all the changes your body is going through and let you know which are flare symptoms and which are just part of being pregnant.

You're going to be in close contact with your doctor, anyway: being pregnant with lupus is a very doctor-intensive nine months. Because you are considered "high risk" (anything beyond normal pregnancy), your physician will want to see you on a regular basis to check your progress and health.

Nutrition and exercise

Eating healthy and exercising in moderation are key to a good pregnancy, and doubly important for someone with lupus. Nutrition for a pregnant woman is covered in many books, so I'm not going to go into detail here. Suffice it to say, you need to eat right, and you need to eat on a regular basis. Skipping meals, bingeing, or eating all Twinkies is right out. If you feel you aren't gaining enough weight to support your baby's needs, or you're gaining too much and are concerned, you need to consult your doctor. Because of your lupus, your physician may have you consult a dietician or nutritionist about neonatal diet.

This isn't the time to say, "I can eat anything I want because I'm pregnant." Being pregnant with lupus is still a risky business, and you need to do everything you can to help your baby. Just about everything that goes into your body can pass through the umbilical cord to the baby; that includes your vitamins, that taco you just ate, and the double espresso you had this morning (and you wondered why the baby was kicking so much!). Neonatal vitamins are probably going to be necessary for you: consult your physician about what is best.

Exercise in moderation is great for a pregnant woman, and especially good for a woman with lupus. Don't stop your exercise regime because you're pregnant. As the pregnancy progresses, you'll find you need to modify your workout; perhaps you'll have to change from a running machine to walking, or from aerobics to yoga. *Whatever you do, check with your doctor before you change or start a new exercise program.* There are great classes especially for pregnant women—check and see if the one that interests you would be appropriate, given your special circumstances with lupus. If you are in a flare, your exercise will need to be modified even more; again, your doctor can help you figure out what's best for you. It may be that gentle stretching and walking every day is going to be best. It may be that you can do a complete gym workout three times a week. Every woman, and every lupus patient, is different.

Reducing stress

Cast your mind back to what you learned in Day Four. What was the key to lowering your chances of a lupus flare? Stress reduction. Less stress equals less flare.

The risk of pregnancy with lupus is your chance for a flare, or flares, during the nine months and the months following your baby's birth. There are certain effects of lupus on pregnancy that you can't do a thing about, such as the risk of blood clots to the placenta, high blood pressure, and premature birth, but you *can* control your risk of many other conditions that can come on via a flare by taking care of your stress.

This means you may have to make compromises in your life while you're pregnant that you might otherwise not have to make if you didn't have lupus. You may have to start working part-time, flexible hours, or even decide that you want to work at home—if that's possible. If your work situation isn't flexible, you may have to look at either moving to another job or even starting a new business that you can run at home. We discussed these types of compromises in Day Four. Make no mistake about it: life with lupus means your life isn't going to be like it was before. Pregnancy doubles that. But if you think it's worthwhile to have a baby, all the compromises in the world will seem to be nothing compared to the joy of your child.

Remember: reduce stress, reduce stress, reduce stress.

Medications and compromises

Another compromise may be what medications you can take while pregnant. Most of the NSAIDs and baby aspirin are safe, and can be used for inflammation reduction. Remember: everything that enters your body has a chance of being passed to the baby through the umbilical cord and placenta. This means you have to be very careful about anything you eat or drink, including your medications.

Your doctor will go over your medications with you and monitor their effect on your blood and other body functions, to make sure both you and baby are healthy. If you develop a flare or need more inflammation reduction than simple nonsteroidal anti-inflammatories can provide, your physician may try the following medications that don't pass through the placenta to the baby:

○ Prednisone
○ Prednisolone
○ Medrol (still debated if this gets through the placenta)

There are several immunosuppressants that have been studied with pregnancy, but the final word isn't in on the following:

o   azathioprine (Imuran)
o   hydroxychloroquine (Plaquenil)

Cytoxan is definitely harmful to a baby, and passes through the placenta easily. If it's used during the first trimester (first three months) of pregnancy, it can harm the baby.

Talk to your doctor before becoming pregnant. Go over all your medications and weed out the harmful ones, substituting others if possible. If you are dependent on medications that can harm a developing baby, you may have to think twice about becoming pregnant. That brings us back to compromise: you may have to make some hard decisions about your health and the health of your baby—that's why planning a pregnancy ahead of time is so important if you have lupus.

IN A SENTENCE:

> *A woman with lupus can have a healthy pregnancy and baby, but compromises will have to be made and the pregnancy will need to be planned for ahead of time.*

learning

Pregnancy & Lupus

WOMEN WITH lupus can and do get pregnant and have healthy babies, though about one quarter (25%) of pregnant women with lupus deliver prematurely due to complications rising from their disease which interact with the pregnancy.

We'll discuss some of the risks of pregnancy with lupus, what can be done to help and treat those risks, and the prognosis for women with lupus who have babies.

What could go wrong?

The primary risk in a lupus pregnancy is premature birth. According to the Lupus Foundation of America, about 25% of all women with lupus who have babies end up with a premature birth. Miscarriages or sudden death of the baby while in utero account for less than 20%. However, the statistics are positive overall: 50% of women with lupus who have babies have a completely normal pregnancy. Compared to only ten years ago, that's a good percentage: up until about a decade ago, women with lupus were discouraged from pregnancy altogether.

FLARES

Some flares will occur during pregnancy. They tend not to be severe and most often involve the usual culprits: fatigue, aches, arthritis, and skin rashes. If a woman becomes pregnant during a flare, she's more likely to have more severe flares during and after her pregnancy than a woman who conceives several months after her latest flare. Some women, for reasons nobody understands, report that they have little or no flares during and after pregnancy, as if being pregnant had put them into remission.

Some doctors will treat a pregnant woman with lupus by giving her Prednisone prophylactically, in a bid to stave off flares during her pregnancy, but there isn't sufficient evidence to prove that this will necessarily work.

TOXEMIA

This form of hypertension (high blood pressure) is also known as pre-eclampsia or pregnancy-induced hypertension. It's not unusual for any woman to develop toxemia during pregnancy, especially during the last trimester; however, women with lupus develop it at a higher than usual percentage: 20% of women with lupus will develop it during pregnancy.

Toxemia includes:

○ high blood pressure, or
○ protein in the urine, or
○ both

It needs to be treated immediately in order to prevent damage to the baby and risk to the mother. Women with lupus may already have kidney disease—accounting for protein in the urine—or high blood pressure, but since toxemia and these conditions are treated in the same manner, there's little difference.

BLOOD CLOTS

About one-third of women with lupus have the antiphospholipid antibodies we discussed in Month Six. These antibodies, including the lupus anticoagulant and anticardiolipin antibody, cause DVTs and blood clots.

Blood clots can form in the placenta, causing miscarriage. They can also block nutrition going to the baby, which means it won't grow as big or as well as it should. Because these clots can form from the second trimester onward, if the clot forms late enough, the baby can be delivered without a problem. However, some women need to be administered with Heparin or baby aspirin to thin the blood enough to prevent or break up clots that may have formed.

Prognosis for a woman who is at risk for blood clots during pregnancy is quite good, if she is given prophylactic medication, such as Heparin: about 80% of those treated have a normal birth and baby.

Neonatal lupus

As we discussed in Day One, there is a form of lupus called *neonatal lupus*. This form occurs only in babies born to mothers who have the anti-Ro or anti-SSA antibody in their blood (the anti-Ro is also the antibody found in those with Sjögren's Syndrome). This form of lupus is not like systemic lupus at all—for one thing, it goes away within a few months of birth.

Signs of neonatal lupus include:

- ○ rash (that goes away)
- ○ blood count anomalies (that go away)
- ○ heart murmur (that doesn't go away, but can be treated)

There is a low percentage of children born with neonatal lupus who develop systemic lupus later in life: most likely they will never trigger the "broken" gene on chromosome 1 that they probably inherited from their mother, which then develops lupus later.

Premature Birth

About one-quarter of women who have lupus end up with premature births. Most of them are due to flares, a blood clot, or other conditions from their lupus.

Because of this, it's recommended that:

○ you get a doctor who knows about lupus & pregnancy, and premature births
○ you see your doctor regularly
○ you have regular checkups and blood screenings
○ you follow your diet & exercise program
○ you take your medications as prescribed
○ you get enough rest & relieve stress in your life
○ you schedule your birth in a regular hospital or clinic (no home-birthing)
○ you schedule your birth in a hospital or clinic that has good premature-baby facilities

Care of your baby

Your baby should be born without any major problems—statistics are on your side with modern medicine and knowledge of lupus. You will want to take care of your baby as a normal mother, but you may need extra help if you have a flare after your pregnancy, or if the birthing process made you go right into a flare.

Lean on your support group during this time. You may want to schedule a relative, best friend, or spouse to come into the house and help take care of the baby so you can rest and get your strength back. You need to take care of *you,* or you won't be able to take care of anything else in the future. Your support group can help with that. Don't be afraid to ask for aid after your pregnancy; people will not only understand, but be willing to do many things for you and your spouse, such as shopping, babysitting, helping clean the house, even taking care of you while your spouse takes care of the baby, or vice versa.

You may want to think about breastfeeding and your situation with lupus. If you are taking medications, most of them can be passed to the baby through your milk, especially corticosteroids like Prednisone, or immunosuppressants such as Imuran or Plaquenil. Talk to your doctor about the possibility of breastfeeding, however, and see what he says.

Also be aware that premature babies usually can't suckle a breast, and even if you can breastfeed, you may have to pump the milk and feed your premature baby through a bottle.

· · ·

Pregnancy used to be discouraged at all costs when it came to women with lupus. Nowadays, many women with lupus not only have a baby, but more than one, and do just fine with it. The process takes planning, scheduling, and compromise, but it can be done.

IN A SENTENCE:

> *Despite the risks, women with lupus can and do have healthy babies if the pregnancy is planned and the woman takes great care with her health during and after the birth.*

Alternative Treatments for Lupus

TRADITIONAL WESTERN, or allopathic, medicine is not alone as a treatment option for lupus patients. More people are supplementing, or turning wholly toward, Eastern, homeopathic, and naturopathic medicines, as well as herbal remedies and homeopathic medicine.

This is not a chapter promoting alternative treatments for lupus, but simply a quick overview of some nonallopathic treatments available to people who would like to explore more medicinal avenues than what their traditional doctor can offer.

Homeopathic medicine

Homeopathic medicine dates from the 1790s, when Dr. Samuel Hahnemann coined the phrase in conjunction with his technique to cure disease by using medicines that would create similar symptoms. In other words, in order to cure the symptoms of a bee sting, one would use bee sting venom—but in microdoses. These doses are referred to as homeopathic doses.

This type of medicine is still practiced by homeopathic doctors, which are more popular in Britain and Europe than in the United States (the royal family of Britain has its own homeopathic doctor). Most people in this country turn to homeopathy as a supplement to, rather than a substitute for, "regular" (allopathic) medicine.

Some conditions stemming from lupus—such as arthritis or tendonitis —may respond to homeopathic medicine, though studies on homeopathic medicine are still debatable and not endorsed by the American Medical Association (AMA), which was the body of physicians largely responsible for discrediting homeopathy after the turn of the twentieth century.

If you go to see a homeopathic doctor, he or she will take a very complete history of your medical symptoms, do a physical examination, and talk to you about your condition. You will be asked things such as "Is the pain burning, stabbing, or throbbing?" and "What would make you feel better when you have (condition): hot or cold?" Hot or cold is one of the base questions in homeopathy, as they feel the body will respond to heat or cold depending on the way disease interacts with your personal body. According to homeopathy, everyone has a different way in which disease affects the body, as the body is not only individually different, but each of us has a spirit or soul inhabiting that body, and so each of us will react to disharmony in the unified field of the body/spirit in a different way. Once the balance is disturbed, disease is created.

Homeopathy is not a licensed practice in the U.S. except in Arizona, Connecticut, and Nevada. There are several institutions that issue certification in homeopathy, but it still remains an unregulated field in the U.S.: anyone, including regular MDs, chiropractors, and laypeople, can claim they are a homeopathic doctor. Check credentials carefully before consultation and *always talk to your regular physician about any medicines you may add to your regime.*

Naturopathy

This variation of alternative medicine is practiced by certified naturopathic doctors, who combine a number of alternative therapies and techniques, including botanical medicine, clinical nutrition, homeopathy,

acupuncture, traditional oriental medicine, hydrotherapy, and naturopathic manipulative therapy. Naturopathic doctors who are also medical doctors use traditional Western medicine and diagnostics, as well
as modern hospital facilities and care standards.

Again, always check with your rheumatologist and/or primary care
physician before adding to or changing any of your treatments or prescribed medicines.

Chiropractic therapy

Many people see chiropractors nowadays: most states license chiropractors as they do doctors, and most health insurance companies have
come to include at least a limited amount of chiropractic coverage in
their policies.

Chiropractic theory is based on the idea that illness comes from
imbalances in the musculoskeletal areas of your body, particularly your
spine, and that by adjusting those areas the body will have the capac-
ity to heal itself. While no empirical evidence has shown that chiropractic treatments can heal chronic diseases such as lupus, someone
suffering from aches and pains of lupus-related conditions may gain
some relief from chiropractic sessions—particularly for mild arthritis,
back pain, and muscle aches.

I broke my back (compression fractures) just before my various syndromes started to surface—in fact, that accident may have been the trigger for them to become active—and once I had healed from the fractures,
I found my continued back pain could be helped with the aid of a local
chiropractor. He has gotten me out of a number of jams (pun intended)
over the years, when my back, ankles, and knees have acted up from
arthritis and general aches. Not once, however, has he claimed he could
heal me of lupus. I am relieved by his honesty.

Herbal medicine

Much has been made of herbal medicines in the last decade, especially for the "natural" treatment of illnesses such as depression. But

little still remains regulated in the herbal medicine market, and so the buyer must continue to beware.

Be careful adding any herbs to your regime: talk to your doctor carefully about anything you may wish to take in any form, be it pill or tea or what-have-you. Herbs *are* medicine: what do you think most medicines are made of? Aspirin is made from the bark of a tree, for instance. Any herb you could add to your diet, as a supplement or a medicine, affects your health. If you'd like to explore taking some herbal remedies for your lupus or conditions related to it, go over a list of what you'd like to take with your doctor before putting anything in your diet. You could, potentially, aggravate your symptoms, unintentionally double up on the effects of a medicine you already take, or even cancel out the effects of one of your medicines. Be careful with herbs—they're "real medicine" in nature's form!

Acupuncture

In this country, acupuncture is finally coming into its own, after several studies have been done recently by the National Institutes of Health (NIH) showing that the practice appears to have beneficial effects on a number of illnesses and conditions, including fibromyalgia, chronic pain, headaches, arthritis, bowel dysfunction, and other syndromes related to lupus. While the NIH still doesn't understand the mechanisms of why acupuncture seems to work the way it does, they do know that it affects certain systems in the body: blood flow to the brain, the immune system, the central nervous system, and blood pressure.

Acupuncture consists of a therapist inserting very thin needles into certain points of the body (acupoints) along the "meridians." These meridians are where traditional Chinese and Oriental medicine say patterns of energy flow—this energy is Qi. When Qi is blocked, disease and pain occur. The needles are left in for a period of time while the patient reclines on a flat surface, and then the needles are removed. Sessions take about an hour each, and most therapists see their clients once a week or more, as needed.

I was personally hesitant about acupuncture for a long time, until it was highly recommended by a friend who swore it wouldn't hurt, and that it was effective for pain from fibromyalgia as well as back pain. Skeptical, I tried it. Either the placebo effect is darned good (in which case, I still don't care—the pain is lessened considerably by treatments), or acupuncture really does work. My pain from fibromyalgia is less than it has been in years, my back is better than its ever been since before I broke it, and my digestive disorder has been under control. I see Jeanne Ann once every two weeks now, and wouldn't hesitate to recommend a lupus patient to give it a try if he or she had chronic pain or fibromyalgia-type pain and conditions. How my immune system has reacted is hard to gauge: I am on immunosuppressant drugs, and without them in the loop, I can't estimate if any changes have occurred since I started acupuncture treatment.

Is it a cure-all? No, I don't think anything is. I, like most people, prefer to seek out those treatments which are beneficial to my personal condition, in a combination that works for me.

Did I seek my doctor's approval before doing anything "alternative," including acupuncture or chiropractic therapy? You bet I did! Never do anything in a vacuum when it comes to your health decisions: you have a chronic disease that your physician is treating. If you don't bring him or her into the loop, you could put your health at risk. Always, always, always talk to your doctor first.

IN A SENTENCE:

> *Many alternative therapies exist for the lupus patient, but you should always seek your doctor's advice before changing any medicines or supplementing your "traditional" treatments.*

learning

Alternative versus Traditional?

WHILE "ALTERNATIVE" medicines and treatments seem to be a new thing or even a fad, many of them have been around a great deal longer than traditional Western allopathic medicine. What will your doctor think if you try something different? How can you talk to your doctor about alternative medicine? What will your friends and family think? What is a gimmick as versus a "real" alternative medicine, and how can you tell the difference? These are some of the questions we'll explore in this Living section.

Finding an alternative doctor or therapist

You may have read an article or heard from a friend about an alternative therapy you'd like to try, but you have no idea where to start.

First of all, talk to your support group about it: many of them may have tried the same therapy or technique, and they may have feedback for you, as well as recommendations about physicians or therapists. Try to get a balanced feel for what you're seeking; read up on the technique on the Net—and not just at places that promote it. Check out articles at the NIH Web site (www.nih.gov) or go to Google (www google.com) and do a search for sites that review therapies with an unbiased approach, such as a university school of medicine or encyclopedia. Ask at your local health food store about alternative therapies and who practices in your area. Most areas of the country have handbooks listing alternative medicinal practices, along with an overview of those techniques and what you can expect from them; your natural food store may have such a book, or it may be in your local library. Ask at the gym, as sometimes alternative practices have links to local area health facilities such as gymnasiums. By all means ask people who have actually been to see the therapist you're investigating. If necessary, ask the therapist if he or she has patient references they can share with you.

Finally, don't forget to talk to your regular doctor about alternative approaches to treating your symptoms, especially for pain control. Most physicians are open to talking about what various therapies can do for lupus patients and their syndromes.

How can I talk to my doctor?

Which brings us to what you may be dreading the most: talking to your doctor about alternative medicine. Most people are scared of bringing up the subject of alternative medicine and therapies with their "regular" physicians. Trust me: it's not as bad as you think.

Most doctors are quite open to talking about alternative medicine and therapies. Many, in fact, have sought out some for themselves, in the form of chiropractic care or acupuncture or even herbal remedies. If your doctor seems as though he or she will be averse to the subject, you may want to sound out your doctor's nurse or physician's assistant first. Ask them what they think your doctor's reaction might be. You may be surprised.

You may want to go about it nonconfrontationally. Don't attack your doctor and say, "You aren't doing me any good with this pain—I want to try acupuncture!" After all, if you have been suffering from chronic pain, your doctor has probably been trying his or her best to alleviate that pain without harm to you. By accusing your doctor of not doing his job, you'll be putting him on the defense, and none of us like being defensive about our work, particularly if we have an ego about it. Instead, try turning the conversation back onto yourself: "I feel as if for some reason I'm not getting the relief I should from the medicine I'm taking. Do you think it could help if I tried acupuncture as a supplement to what you're doing for me? I've investigated it a bit, and I think it may be a good technique for my particular condition. What do you think?"

Try engaging your physician in an adult-to-adult discussion about your health care in a similar manner whenever you want to talk about alternatives or changes to your treatment. It may do a world of good in your relationship.

What will my friends and family think?

If you have friends like mine, they'll be supportive in just about any decision you make about your health care. But some people find that exploring alternative medicine puts them on the defensive with the ones around them; many people don't approve of therapies other than the ones with which they're familiar.

What's the cure? Education, put simply. Place articles about the therapy you're using in their hands; send them articles from reputable Internet sites, such as universities or the NIH; give them pamphlets provided by your therapist or alternative doctor.

Or, take them along for a visit. My husband was supportive, but unsure, of my use of acupuncture—plus, I needed the ride—and so I took him with me to the acupuncturist. He watched a session, talked to me while I was on the table with the needles in, and generally got himself comfortable with the technique. Now he goes with me on a regular basis, but usually takes a nap on the couch in the treatment room while I am "needled." He seems very comfortable with the technique now!

Remember, the bottom line is that it's your body, your health, and your health care. *You* need to be the person who is comfortable with your alternative doctor or therapist, and with the alternative medicine you've chosen. It's good to have the support of your friends and family, but sometimes you can't please all of the people all of the time. Don't let someone's misunderstanding of an educated choice you've made be a detriment to the health care you could receive.

How can I tell if something's a gimmick or scam?

Good question, and one that's not always easy to answer.

In general, you can smell a gimmick or fad by its newness, or by its snake-oil factor. For "newness," in other words, is this something that is just out on the market and remains unproven, but everyone seems to be talking about it? Does it cost more than its older alternative but with no *empirical* proven improvement? (I'm thinking of "coral calcium" as versus regular calcium, for instance—one of the current gimmicks on the health food market.)

When I say "snake oil" I'm referring to the old-fashioned snake-oil salesman kind of gimmick: once a snake oil, always a snake oil—it doesn't matter that the old carnies are gone and such cure-alls aren't sold from behind the tent of a circus show anymore. The same old song and dance still goes on. Does the product claim to improve or even cure all sorts of completely unrelated (medical) conditions? I smell snake oil, then. Or, as a friend of mine often says, "If it's really too good to be true, then it probably ain't true."

Sometimes a product or therapy will come onto the market and be so new and so good that it appears to be a gimmick or a new version of an older snake oil, and yet after some time and some empirical analysis by standardized modern medicine, said product or technique will prove to be valid. You just never know. Unfortunately, you can't tell gimmick or scam from good product sometimes, and only time will tell.

In general, follow my friend's rule of thumb, and if some therapy or medicine claims to be "too good," run—don't walk—away from it. Not everything is perfect, even standard Western medicine. Anything that claims to be otherwise is just so much snake oil.

. . .

Finally, you may ask if your insurance company will cover health costs related to alternative medicines and therapies. Some do, some don't. Some cover particular medicines, some don't. All you can do is ask your insurance carrier or health coverage provider about what various medicines and therapies will be covered and in what amounts (pay special attention to amounts: many will cover therapies such as chiropractic visits, but only for so many sessions per year, per incident).

Every year more "alternative" therapies come under coverage with health insurance companies as more empirical evidence shows certain techniques to have valid applications in medicine. Keep checking with your health insurance to see what they cover.

IN A SENTENCE:

> *Finding an alternative doctor or therapist, talking to your regular doctor, and educating your support system about alternative medicine may be easier than you think—you may want to give it a try.*

Lupus Research and the Future

LUPUS USED to be a mostly fatal disease, because it was diagnosed so late in its progression. Now, with better and faster diagnostics, a person with lupus can live a long life. In the future, we may be able to look for a cure of the disease, but first medical research needs to be completed on finding out what exactly causes lupus.

A brief history of lupus research

A historical outlook of lupus is an odd thing to have at the end of a book, but if we don't look at where we have been, it's hard to plot a course for where we're going in the future.

The first descriptions of lupus as a unique disease were made by a physician named Rogerius in the thirteenth century. He described the facial lesions caused by lupus masking as like "a wolf bite" and named the syndrome lupus after the Latin word for *wolf*. More observations of facial discoid lupus were made throughout the nineteenth century, but in 1872, Kaposi first described the systemic nature of the disease:

... lupus erythematosus ... may be attended by altogether more severe pathological changes ... and even dangerous constitutional symptoms may be intimately associated with the process in question, and that death may result from conditions which must be considered to arise from the local malady. (Kaposi MN. "Neue Beitrage zur Keantiss des lupus erthematosus." *Arch Dermatol Syphilol* 1872; 4:36.)

By 1904, a full description of both the systemic nature of lupus and its discoid cousin were observed and described. In 1948, Hargraves discovered the LE cell, which changed the nature of how lupus was observed and brought it fully into twentieth-century medicine—because of the LE cell's involvement with lupus, suddenly medical practitioners were aware that lupus was an autoimmune disease. This is also the period when the false-syphilis test was first recognized as an indicator for lupus. In the fifties, both animal models of lupus were studied and a breakthrough involving twins showed a genetic link in lupus: a predisposition in genetic markers.

Lupus is now classified as a rheumatological inflammatory disease which is also an autoimmune disease. There is clearly a predisposition in known genetic markers on chromosome 1, but that's about as far as medical science has gone thus far. As of 2003, the human genome project is "complete": the genetic code—as we understand it—for the human race has been catalogued, but you need to realize that having a map doesn't mean you know what the roads really do and where they go. Decades of work still needs to be done in individual fields of study to find out what genes "do" what. As of now, no one *really* knows what causes lupus, what may trigger it in some but not in others, and there is no known cure.

What does the future hold?

Just about every day I read articles that detail a breakthrough or discovery in medical science: we live in Interesting Times, indeed. Even as I wrote this book, discoveries were made in the field of lupus research about genetic markers, chromosomal interactions, and treatments for similar autoimmune or rheumatological diseases that may, in the future, also be applied to lupus.

Gene therapy used to be a science-fiction trope; now it is a reality (though still highly experimental). Soon we may all have access to gene therapy for diseases we carry, dormant, in our genetic code. Beyond that, we may even have gene therapy for diseases that are active in our bodies—such as lupus. And I'm talking about *in our lifetimes,* if medical research continues to receive the funding it needs to further its work.

Get involved. Contribute to foundations and clinics that perform research on lupus and other rheumatological diseases. Join the Lupus Foundation of America or your local lupus chapter: get the word out to your friends that these foundations need their support as well. Without grassroots efforts, many of the breakthroughs that have taken place lately would never have happened, what with national funding cut to much of the sciences, including the NIH.

It's up to you and me and everyone we know to keep lupus in the forefront of people's minds. This isn't just an obscure "women's disease"; it affects over one million Americans and millions of others throughout the world, many of whom suffer the disease without a diagnosis. We need to make sure everyone knows what lupus is, what it can do, and how they can help us find a cure.

IN A SENTENCE:

> *Lupus has been misunderstood for many years, but it's up to us to educate the public and our friends on how to help us find a cure for it.*

living

Your Life with Lupus

BY NOW you've lived a full year after receiving the diagnosis that you have systemic lupus. You have learned much, experienced much, and have been down many roads on your journey toward living with a chronic disease. Now it's time to look at the future and what it holds for you, both in how you will live your life with lupus always by your side, and how the future bodes for you and for all those who have this disease.

Moving on

During the first weeks after diagnosis, you learned that lupus, like all chronic diseases, brings with it the emotions and rationalizations of grief and bereavement. You felt denial, anger, sadness, and finally acceptance about your diagnosis of lupus. You learned that cycles of these stages of grief will continue throughout your life, as the disease will never really go away; as it comes and goes with flares and remissions, you may experience some or all of these feelings again and again, in differing degrees.

Now it's time to think about the future. How are you going to get on with your life? Are you going to stay bound to a fear that lupus will rule your life, with its flares and remissions, forever? Or are you going to realize that, as with anything in life, your chronic disease is something that *is* within your control—as much as we control anything in this crazy world. Sure, you're going to get sick again—that's a given if you have lupus, unless you're one of those extraordinary, one-in-a-million individuals who go into remission and never have a relapse in their lives. Okay, so you get sick again. You could also be hit by a car tomorrow on your way to the subway station. Is that going to keep you from walking out your front door for the rest of your life? The same goes for your lupus: you have to go on. You can't just *stop* because you have a chronic disease.

AA (Alcoholics Anonymous) coined the phrase, "One day at a time." That's very apt for all of us. We really can only take life one day at a time—plans are always going to fall through, rain is always going to come unexpectedly on the day of your daughter's outdoor wedding, and that concert you were waiting to go see since 1990 is going to get cancelled at the last minute. Such things happen. Good things happen, too—usually more than the bad. All you can do is make the best plans you can for the future and hope for the best. If a flare comes up, you'll deal with it when it does. If you end up in the hospital with pericarditis, it's not going to be much fun while you have it, but then you'll most likely get over it in a few weeks, and make plans all over again.

Moving on means *moving forward*.

Taking responsibility

When you have a chronic disease, it's easy to become dependent on others. After all, some of the time you really *will* be dependent on others for your health care, your daily needs, and your support. You won't always be able to do everything for yourself when you're sick with lupus: you'll need others to pick up your medications, take you to the doctor, and help take care of the cats. But that doesn't mean you aren't responsible for yourself anymore.

You need to remember that you're in charge of your life, still, no matter how sick you get. You are responsible to make sure you get proper medical attention. Remember how we discussed in Week Three that it's critical for you to remember that you need to keep your doctor aware of your needs? And that if you aren't satisfied with your medical care, you need to pursue that yourself? It's *your* health, *your* health care, and in the end, the doctor works for *you*.

You need to be responsible for taking your medications: no one can force pills down your throat (okay, they *can*, if they're Nurse Rackett, but it's easier if you take them yourself!). You're the one in charge of making sure you keep on schedule with your prescriptions and take them all every day, according to your doctor's orders. Do the adult thing and organize your medications in whatever method suits you best, as we discussed in Week Two. It's hard to do sometimes, and sometimes you'll need someone from your support group to help you. At the beginning it's particularly hard, but by now—a full year later—you need to *move on* and take responsibility for yourself—when you're well enough to do so, of course.

Planning for the future

Finally, you need to look toward the future. You do have one, after all. Having a chronic disease is not the same thing as having a fatal disease. You have a future, and you need to start planning for it—*with* lupus.

You will most likely live a full life with lupus, as I said during Week One. Most lupus patients live to a ripe old age, or die of a completely unrelated disease or accident. Since no one can plan ahead for an accident, you may as well plan for a long life.

"But I'll have a chronic disease all that time!" you might be whining. Stop whining for a minute and listen to Nancy: she's about to be mean to you. *So you have a chronic disease: tough noogies.* You don't have anything that will necessarily kill you right off the bat; you don't have anything that will necessarily make you go butt-ugly; and you don't have anything that will make the neighbors move away in horror and fear of contagion. There are many worse things to contract than lupus. Sure, it's not a great disease to have, and having a chronic disease is a real pain in the butt to have in the first place. But you *will have a life,* even if it's a life with lupus.

I know I'm sounding like a tough-girl version of Pollyanna here, but after many years with fibromyalgia, Sjögren's Syndrome, Raynaud's Syndrome, and being diagnosed (and undiagnosed, and rediagnosed, and undiagnosed again) with lupus, I can say from experience that as chronic diseases go, lupus isn't so very bad. Not compared to some others I've experienced firsthand: for instance, my mother died of adult-onset multiple sclerosis. I count my blessings that I don't have that. Same goes for the cancer that killed my stepfather. I could go on and on, ad nauseam, but I'm sure you get the point (and that you have your own stories you could fill in here).

I'm not being unsympathetic to those with lupus who have severe systemic lupus, and those who have almost continual flares. There are people who are *very* sick with lupus, don't get me wrong. And I'm not downplaying that at all. What I am saying is that *most* people with lupus live through flares *and* remissions, and live full lives in between the flares.

After all, isn't that what most of life is? Life between the flares of other things that get in the way of the good stuff, the fun stuff, the stuff that makes us smile. It's the life *in between* that we need to aim for, and to plan for. That's the future of living with lupus.

IN A SENTENCE:

> *You can live a full life with lupus, even though you have a chronic disease—just give yourself the chance to look beyond your disease and plan for the future.*

ACETAMINOPHEN—a pain reliever, such as Tylenol

ADVANCE DIRECTIVE—a legal document that dictates your pre-ferred medical care in case of incapacity and/or a vegetative state. These can be created and filed at any local hospital or home health care facility.

ANEMIA—low red blood cell count

ANTI-INFLAMMATORIES—medicines that reduce inflammation in the body

ANTICARDIOLPIN ANTIBODY—these autoimmune antibodies are part of a spectrum known as antiphospholipid antibody syndrome (APS). (See antiphosopholipid.)

ANTIMALARIAL—a drug that is taken to prevent malaria; it is also used widely in treating rheumatoid arthritis diseases, including lupus and some of its overlapping syndromes.

ANTIPHOSPHOLIPID ANTIBODY—the autoantibodies that can cause blood clots

AUTOANTIBODY—an antibody involved in immune reactions; an antibody that reacts against the tissues of the body that created it.

AUTOIMMUNE DISEASE—a disease which affects the immune system of the body, that which keeps you protected from illness and disease

BIOFEEDBACK—a technique that utilizes a device that records your brain activity and autonomic responses; you learn to control your responses by paying attention to what the device tells you your body is doing

BOARD CERTIFIED—certification in a particular specialty given by the AMA

BUTTERFLY RASH—see "lupus mask"

CHRONIC FATIGUE SYNDROME (CFS)—a syndrome which causes unexplained, overwhelming fatigue; it is often carried with fibromyalgia

CLINICAL CHRONIC FATIGUE—fatigue that is overwhelming, persistent (chronic), not related to any sleep disorder, and is clinically diagnosed

COGNITIVE DYSFUNCTION—any dysfunction that affects the mind, memory, thinking faculties

CONNECTIVE TISSUE—all tissue within the body that connects to bone or cartilage

CORTICOSTEROID—a form of steroid that reduces inflammation in the body

CUTANEOUS LUPUS (see discoid lupus)

DISCOID LUPUS—a form of lupus which primarily affects the skin

DRUG-INDUCED LUPUS—a form of lupus caused by a medicine

EMBOLUS—when a piece of a blood clot breaks off and travels in the body along a vein

FALSE-POSITIVE SYPHILIS TEST—a false reading of positive for syphilis that shows up in many lupus patients

FIBROMYALGIA—a rheumatological syndrome which causes pain throughout the body, particularly in certain "trigger points"; it can also cause fatigue and symptoms similar to lupus

FLARE—when lupus is active and you can get sick

HEMOSTASIS—thickening or coagulation of blood

IBUPROFEN—an NSAID, such as Advil

IMMUNOSUPPRESSANT—a drug that suppresses the immune system's responses

INTERNIST—a doctor who specializes in internal medicine; is usually board certified

IRRITABLE BOWEL SYNDROME (IBS)—a syndrome in which the bowel is inflamed and dysfunctional; often associated with fibromyalgia

KETOSIS—protein spilling into the urine

LEUKOPENIA—low white blood cell count

LUPUS ANTICOAGULANT FACTOR—one of the antiphospholipid antibodies, which can cause blood clots

LUPUS FOG—a cognitive dysfunction that occurs in lupus patients, causing memory loss, confusion, fatigue, and clumsiness

LUPUS MASK—the butterfly rash which typifies discoid lupus; also called the malar rash, butterfly rash, or wolf's mask

LUPUS NEPHRITIS—kidney disease in lupus patients

MALAR RASH—the clinical term for the lupus mask; see "lupus mask"

MEDICAL POWER OF ATTORNEY—a legal document giving someone power to make medical decisions in case the patient is unable to do so herself

MEDROL—a corticosteroid drug

MYOFASCIA—the connecting tissue between the organs and other parts of your body that don't have muscle, bone, or organ—sort of like packing material in the spaces of your body

MYOFASCIAL PAIN SYNDROME (MPS)—a syndrome wherein the myofascia are inflamed; similar in many ways to fibromyalgia

NEUTROPENIA—low granulocytes count

NSAIDs—nonsteroidal anti-inflammatories, such as Celebrex or Advil

OVERLAPPING LUPUS—a form of lupus which includes other syndromes

PATIENT ADVOCATE—someone who helps a patient with communication between the patient and doctor

PERICARDIAL EFFUSION—liquid in the lining surrounding the heart

PERICARDITIS—an inflammation of the lining surrounding the heart

PLAQUENIL—hydroxychloroquine, an antimalarial drug used to treat rheumatological diseases and their symptoms; also used to treat chronic fatigue

PLEURAL EFFUSION—liquid in the pleural lining of the chest wall, around the lungs

PLEURAL LINING—the lining surrounding the lungs

PLEURISY—an inflammation of the lining surrounding the lungs (pleural lining)

PLEURITIS—another name for pleural effusion

PNEUMONIA—liquid in the lungs

POSTPHLEBITIC SYNDROME, or **PHLEBITIS**—a syndrome that can occur after a DVT, where the veins in the affected limb tend to dysfunction, causing pain

PREDNISONE—a corticosteroid often used to treat lupus and other inflammatory conditions

PULMONARY SYSTEM—the system in the body which includes the lungs and circulatory system

RAYNAUD'S SYNDROME—a rheumatological syndrome which affects the capillary action in the body, particularly in the hands and feet

REMISSION—when lupus isn't active and you don't necessarily get sick

RHEUMATOLOGICAL DISEASE—disease which affects systems of the muscles and joints, causing pain; also, any disease that's classified with rheumatoid arthritis

RHEUMATOLOGIST—a doctor who specializes in rheumatology, which includes lupus

ROSACEA—a skin condition which affects the capillaries in the face, causing redness and a type of acne

SJÖGREN'S SYNDROME—a rheumatological syndrome which primarily affects the formation of saliva and tear film, but which can also act exactly like lupus, with connective tissue affected throughout the body

SPECIALISTS—doctors who specialize in a particular field of medicine; most are board-certified by the American Medical Association (AMA) in their specialty

SUBCUTANEOUS—under the skin (subcutaneous injection goes under the skin)

THROMBOLUS—a blood clot

VASCULITIS—blood vessels in the body become inflamed

WOMAN'S DISEASE—diseases affecting primarily women; also, diseases which doctors feel may be primarily psychosomatic

For Further Information

American Medical Association (AMA) information on advance directives Web site: http://www.ama-assn.org/public/booklets/livgwill.htm

Arthritis Foundation Web site: http://www.arthritis.org

Bedsock knitting pattern: Nancy C. Hanger, windhaven@mac.com

Cilley, Martha (the Fly Lady). *Sink Reflections*. Bantam Doubleday Dell: New York, 2002. Also see the FlyLady's Web site, where you can sign up for her system for free: http://www.flylady.com. (This is the best system I've ever seen for people who need organization in very little time each time—perfect for people who are chronically ill. It can be applied to anything, not just cleaning your house.)

FDA Food Pyramid Web site brochure: http://www.pueblo.gsa.gov/cic_text/food-pyramid/main.htm

Lupus Foundation of America articles: http://www.lupus.org/education/articles.html

Lupus Foundation of America informational brochures: http://www.lupus.org/education/brochures.html

National Diabetes Information Clearinghouse, "What I Need to Know About Eating and Diabetes": http://diabetes.niddk.nih.gov/dm/pubs/eating_ez/index.htm

National Institutes of Health (NIH) information on durable medical power of attorney Web site: http://www.nlm.nih.gov/medlineplus/ency/article/001908.htm

National Institutes of Health—National Institute of Arthritis and Musculoskeletal and Skin Diseases Web site: http://www.nih.gov/niams/

National Institutes of Health, Fibromyalgia information Web site: http://
www.nih.gov/niams/healthinfo/fibrofs.htm

National Institutes of Health, Special Diets for Special Needs: http://rex.nci.
nih.gov/NCI_Pub_Interface/Eating_Hints/eatdiets.html

National Women's Health Resource Center at iVillage Women's Health:
http://www.ivillagehealth.com/library/nwh

Nielsen Hayden, Teresa. *Making Book.* NESFA Press, 2nd ed. 1996. ($11.00
+ $2 shipping, the NESFA Press, PO Box 809, Framingham, MA 01701-
0203)

St. Thomas' Hospital, London, "Lupus Patients Understanding and Support"
Web site: http://www.lupus-support.org.uk (information therein based on
Understanding Lupus by Dr. Graham Hughes, head of the Lupus Research
Unit at St. Thomas' Hospital—this Web site is where an alternative check-
list of lupus symptoms can be found).

Starlanyl, Devin, M.D. and Mary Ellen Copeland. *Fibromyalgia & Chronic
Myofascial Pain Syndrome: A Survival Manual.* New Harbingers Publica-
tions, Inc.: Oakland, CA, 1996.

Van Vorous, Heather. *The First Year—IBS.* Marlowe & Company: New York,
2001. Also, http://www.eatingforibs.com

V.I.A.L. of LIFE Web site information (Note: requires Acrobat reader for your
computer, which can be downloaded free from Adobe at http://www.
adobe.com) : http://www.sjfd.com/vial_of_life.pdf

WebMD Web site, for reliable generalized medical information in abstracts
and full article form: http://www.webmd.com

Organizations:

Lupus Foundation of America, Inc.
1300 Piccard Drive, Suite 200
Rockville, MD 20850-4303
Phone: (301) 670-9292 9 AM–5 PM (ET) Monday-Friday
Fax: (301) 670-9486
1-800-558-0121 (Information request line)
1-800-558-0231 (Para información en Español)

Acknowledgments

Thanks go to the many people who have helped me through this project, putting up with a cranky author at all hours of the day and night:

James D. Macdonald, NR-WEMT-I, for his expertise in writing and emergency medicine information; the Wolfbytes mailing list, for their support and always-informative discussions, as well as late-night conversations; Modean Moon, for her insight; Teresa Nielsen Hayden, for her marvelous prose; Bruce Hadley, for asking me—daily—"aren't you supposed to be writing?"; to Jeanne Ann Whittington, for keeping body and soul pinned together; for the regulars at T.R. Brennan's, for good conversation and all the laughs to get me through this—particularly Brian, for the great martinis; for all the Baen Books people, particularly Jim Baen, for giving me the time and space to write this book; for my agent, Deirdre, for being saintlike; for my editor, Matthew, for patience beyond the call of duty; and for Dr. Andrea Schneebaum, M.D., for her wisdom, laughter, medical knowledge, and a doctor's care that one rarely sees anymore.

Index